Improving Health Services

Improving Health Services

Background, Method and Applications

Walter Holland

London School of Economics and Political Science, UK

Edward Elgar

Cheltenham, UK • Northampton, MA, USA

Published by
Edward Elgar Publishing Limited
The Lypiatts
15 Lansdown Road
Cheltenham
Glos GL50 2JA
UK

Edward Elgar Publishing, Inc.
William Pratt House
9 Dewey Court
Northampton
Massachusetts 01060
USA

A catalogue record for this book
is available from the British Library

Library of Congress Control Number: 2013942243

This book is available electronically in the ElgarOnline.com Social and Political Science Subject Collection, E-ISBN 978 1 78347 019 8

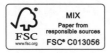

ISBN 978 1 78347 018 1

Typeset by Columns Design XML Ltd, Reading
Printed and bound in Great Britain by T.J. International Ltd, Padstow

Contents

Preface

Health services research is the systematic study of the means by which basic medical and other relevant knowledge is brought to bear on the health of individuals and communities under a given set of conditions.[1]

This is a personal account of the development of health services research (HSR), mainly in the United Kingdom but with reference also to developments in the United States.

I had originally intended to describe and assess all the HSR that had been commissioned and published in the UK but a survey of the available literature revealed three fairly major obstacles to this approach. First, it was not always possible to be sure that projects started had ever been completed and findings published. Second, in some cases I was unable to determine why a study had been commissioned, what problems arose during its execution, and what action if any had been taken as a result. Third, HSR studies in areas other than my own – for example, nursing or dentistry – lay outside my field of expertise so that any conclusions could be open to challenge.

I, therefore, decided to base the book on my own personal experience since this type of research began in the UK in 1962. This has enabled me to describe the background, commissioning and outcome of HSR studies in the particular context of epidemiology. It has meant that there is considerable disparity in the length of some of the chapters. Chapter 5, for example, is very short but requires to stand alone on the central issues of organisation and funding. Chapter 6, in contrast, is very long but once again, since it describes the body of work carried out in the St Thomas' Social Medicine and Health Services Research Unit, it does need to be read as a whole. A note on the text: throughout the text discussion the term Department of Health is often used to describe what was formerly and variously known as the Ministry of Health or the Department of Health and Social Security (DHSS).

Sound HSR is absolutely central to the effective functioning of any modern health service. I hope this book will show how HSR in the UK has developed over time and how it can illuminate and improve health service policy and practice.

REFERENCE

1. Global Advisory Committee on Medical Research (1983). *Who Chronicle*, 37(1), 4–5.

Acknowledgements

This book would not have been possible without the help and encouragement of Professor Elias Mossialos. The facilities at LSE Health and Social Care have enabled the work to be done, particularly the unstinting help of Champa Heidbrink and Naho Ollason. Dr Saka Omer provided expert guidance on the translation of expenditure to current day values. I am most grateful for the advice and discussions with Dr Michael Ashley Miller, Professor Nick Black, Sir Ian Chalmers, Professor Shah Ebrahim, Professor John Grimley Evans, Professor Alan Maynard, Professor Martin McKee, Professor Klim McPherson, Professor Tom Meade, Dr Jeremy Metters, Sir Muir Grey, and Dr Adrian Peatfield. Their views and perspectives have been helpful in sharpening some of my descriptions and opinions. I am also deeply indebted to Professor Charles Florey who has kindly read and commented on the manuscript and corrected some of my most egregious errors and to Mrs Susie Stewart who has undertaken rigorous editing on my behalf and pulled the book into shape.

Of course the greatest gratitude is due to members of the St Thomas' Social Medicine and Health Services Research Unit without whom none of this would have been possible.

1. Health services research: a general perspective

INTRODUCTION

Health services research (HSR) differs markedly from the clinical research traditionally associated with medicine. Most clinical research focuses on the investigation of natural diseases occurring in humans. The problems examined are those posed by knowledge of the normal or diseased and examination occurs within the defined boundaries of a particular branch of science such as genetics, molecular biology or immunology. In clinical research, the main area of enquiry relates to the application of this type of scientific biology to the manifestation and treatment of disease in man and is now often referred to as translational research.

The term HSR is used variably by different groups and is often misunderstood. It describes a field of enquiry characterised by its applied and multidisciplinary nature and occupies territory that includes public health research, population health sciences, health systems research and clinical research. Definitions have been proposed by various organisations and individuals ranging from the Advisory Committee on Medical Research of the World Health Organisation,[1] Flook and Sanazaro,[2] and the Academy of Medical Science Working Group.[3] All are agreed that HSR is concerned with the relationship between need, demand, supply, use and outcome of health services. The discipline, therefore, examines some or all of the following factors: quality, distribution, access, outcome and effectiveness of health care services, irrespective of who provides them.

The tasks of HSR can be categorised under the following four headings:

1. Availability, distribution and use of health care services
    In any health care system, the resources available for health care provision must be defined and examined. This may involve studies of health personnel and the identification of areas of manpower

needs. The distribution of physical resources and personnel must be understood.

2.   Operational characteristics of health care provision
      One of the most important areas covered by HSR is the actual delivery of health care. This may include the description or measurement of work patterns in clinics; determination of transport requirements for patients; assessment of the need for various types of facilities, such as operating theatres; or the development of a rationale for allocating resources between different geographical or social subgroups. This may vary in complexity from simple work studies to complex manpower or economic computer modelling of the whole health care sector.

3.   Determination of attitudes and behaviour
      Consumers of health care services – both therapeutic and preventive – are not passive in their response to the provision of services. Cultural, social and educational factors determine the attitudes of a population to illness and to usage and expectations of health care services. It is necessary, therefore, to understand and measure such factors and this kind of knowledge is of particular importance in planning and mounting public health initiatives.

4.   Technical and economic assessment of the efficacy of medical therapy or technology
      In the past 50 years, there has been a marked growth in technical medicine and it has become economically and functionally essential to measure the technical performance of alternative techniques or strategies in the provision of health services. Such assessment has become the concern not only of the medical profession, but also of the funders and administrators of health care. Assessment may be needed for different patterns of care, exploring alternatives to hospital admission – for example, community care – or to provide a sound social, biological or economic basis for introducing mass immunisation or screening programmes. Problems in arriving at acceptable programmes may arise from biological, behavioural or economic factors and thus this research is likely to extend beyond the relatively simple area of pure biological research. In addition, it may be necessary to look at a new programme in practice before assessment is possible. This type of enquiry is called intervention research and requires the development of pilot studies in order to assess a programme's potential value and cost before wider intro- duction is considered. The aim must be to improve the quality of care but costs in relation to marginal improvements must also be taken into account. Thus, in order to provide appropriate services,

HSR overlaps with epidemiological research since knowledge of the causes, distribution, prevalence and incidence of disease is essential.

The aim of this book is to cover all these fields and to trace the development of HSR in the UK.[i] A brief description of developments in the US is also given to demonstrate the similarities and differences (see Chapter 2).

HISTORICAL BACKGROUND

There is a long history of research into the manifestation and treatment of illness, but the recognition of the importance of HSR as a discrete and necessary component for the adequate functioning of health services on which this treatment depends has been slow to develop. Only in the past 50 years has there been any concerted attempt to coordinate and foster HSR in the UK. There are a number of reasons for this neglect. Probably the most important of these has been the belief that advances in medical treatment and technology are infinite, and that the development of appropriate methods of treatment will solve the majority of ills. This can be well illustrated by the erroneous belief of many of the founders of the National Health Service (NHS) that expenditure on health services would diminish because the introduction of universal services would improve the health of the population and thus lead to lower demand for health services. There is now an appreciation that this is not the case and that the evaluation of health services and what they have to offer is vital if there is to be any reasonable allocation of resources to the health sector by government or society.

The longest history of support for HSR as a distinct entity has been in the US.[4] In 1966 Anderson[5] stated: 'systematic research on health care emerged in the 1920s in response to concerns about equity of access to health services and its emphases have historically selected prevailing societal definitions of the issues surrounding the organisation, financing and quality of health services.'

It is possible to identify four distinct stages in the development of HSR in the US. The first stage, up to the middle of the 1930s, was sporadic and largely descriptive, sponsored by private philanthropic foundations and only rarely covered by governmental funding. During this period, the

---

i. Most of the descriptions are based on the experience in England and Wales during the years 1960–1995.

US Public Health Service began to be concerned with the health of the poor and indigent, in particular with the care of children. A number of largely descriptive studies were started – for example, the community studies in Hagerstown, Maryland.[6]

In the second stage, between 1930 and 1950, the major emphasis was on a national health service, partly to evaluate the effects of the enactment of the Social Security Act and also because of concerns with the performance of the different component parts of the private health sector. Most of the research at this time was undertaken by individuals employed by government agencies, and occasionally by staff financed by private foundations.

It was the third stage – between the 1950s and the mid-1960s – that saw the greatest expansion in HSR as academic institutions gradually became involved. Some of the impetus for this sprang from the availability of repeated national health surveys, the increasing interest of social scientists, the factors governing the use of health services, and the allocation of resources for building hospitals and health facilities. University programmes in health administration began to be introduced and the teaching of community medicine and epidemiology became concerned with matters beyond infectious disease.

In the fourth stage, from the mid-1960s onwards, HSR in the US developed its major strength with the founding of the National Center for Health Services Research and Development, which changed its name several times. There has been an increasing realisation of the need to study the wider problems of health care delivery because of the rising costs of health care and the limits to what clinical medicine can achieve. The subject has been under increasing strain because of the growing complexity of the research required, as well as its far-reaching consequences. It has been well summarised up to the middle of the 1970s by Flook and Sanazaro.[2] More recently, White has described the developments of HSR in the US,[7, 8] and he and Eisenberg give a good account of how HSR can contribute to the development and operation of a market-orientated health care system.[9]

In the UK, six main factors have made the development and support of HSR a necessity.

- Reassessment of the medical task and the role of general economic and social forces in the health status of populations.
- Phenomenal growth in medical manpower and medical technology.
- Rising costs and complexity of health care provision.
- Political and social need for equity of health care provision.
- General increase in the complexity of society and the increasing

scale of social and health effects possible from modern political, environmental and industrial developments.

● Increasing knowledge and expectations of consumers of health care services, through newspaper articles, television and the Internet.

In the last 70 years there has been a gradual reappraisal of the task of medicine and the health care services in the developed world. During a period of phenomenal growth in health care resources, personnel and technology, it has become clear that massive investment in personal health care services has substantial limitations in improving the health and well-being of people, while the potential cost of providing these services is almost limitless. The same period has witnessed the success of public health measures such as immunisation and malaria control. It has been increasingly realised that improvements in diet, water supply, social environment and public awareness may be of far greater importance for the health and welfare of populations than any direct, curative interventions by medical or allied professional staff.

Throughout this period, governments have become more involved, directly or indirectly, in meeting the costs and assisting in the organisation of the national health care system. The increasing political desirability of ensuring equality of access to medical services has followed from this and in turn has raised the general level of demand for and usage of health care services. The last six decades have also seen a rapidly changing environment associated with massive technological innovation. The health outcomes of industrialisation have produced serious social, medical and cultural problems.[10] Against this background, the need for the continual assessment of health care provision, relevance and effectiveness has never been greater and it is in this context that HSR has come of age.

THE ROLE OF HEALTH SERVICES RESEARCH

The role of HSR is to provide evidence on which decision-makers can base their policies and to give managers the technical knowledge to translate these policies into action. This is of profound importance to the well-being of people served by the health care system and there must be a direct link between health care policy and the direction of much of the research being undertaken. But problems arise when issues cross boundaries and are not purely a matter of health. One clear example of this is cigarette smoking, unambiguously recognised as harmful to health. The threefold aim must be to try to persuade individuals not to start smoking in childhood, to produce less harmful smoking products, and to dissuade people from continuing to smoke. From the point of view of the national economy, however, tobacco is a potent source of tax revenue. This is a classic example of the conflict that can arise between different sectors of the national economy; in this case, between the health service and other government departments such as HM Treasury.

Another example of such conflict is seen in the area of industrial development. Coal is a cheap form of energy, but inefficient burning of coal generates a variety of harmful by-products such as suspended particulates, sulphur dioxide (SO_2), nitrogen dioxide (NO_2) and perhaps even carcinogens. Burning coal efficiently prevents atmospheric pollution but increases the cost of production. The hazards of coal burning have been assessed and described by Holland and colleagues.[11] In the national context, however, the benefits to be gained by reducing pollution have to be balanced against the costs incurred.

HSR can provide guidance to policy-makers, managers and providers of health care in two main ways. First, it can evaluate existing or proposed health care measures – evaluation research. Second, it can look at the effect on society of existing or proposed policy measures so that effective health care policy options can be developed – health care research and health policy analysis.

Evaluation Research

Although there is a long history of the technical evaluation of medical care, the use of statistical or epidemiological analysis as a major tool of medical research is comparatively recent. In clinical research, the effectiveness of treatment is seen mainly in purely physiological terms – for example, lowering of blood pressure – or in terms of patient survival – for example, in the assessment of cancer therapy. When considering the effectiveness of a particular drug or other intervention, however, other factors must also be considered. It may be, for example, that complex and costly treatments are best provided from a few specialist centres of excellence. But then patients may be reluctant or unable to travel to such centres that may be some distance from their homes and this may increase geographical health inequalities. A particular intervention required may also be unacceptable to particular social, ethnic or cultural groups and may need to be adapted to meet their requirements – for example, the necessity for gynaecological treatment to be administered by women for some ethnic or religious groups.

The approach of the clinical scientist cannot provide guidance in these areas. In many cases, the purely scientific basis for choosing a particular treatment programme has not yet been satisfactorily resolved. Thus, after almost one century of debate, we still remain unclear as to the best ways of preventing and treating breast cancer.

Decision-makers in any health care planning organisation must take decisions about implementing programmes of care or about determining priorities involving medical, technical, demographic, social, anthropological or economic factors. It is in this context that HSR must operate to evaluate the need for and effectiveness of medical therapies. This can be illustrated by looking at research on preventive procedures such as Lechat's classic study of rubella prevention.[12] The risk of a woman contracting rubella during pregnancy as a cause of malformations in her newborn baby was first observed in Australia in 1941. Lechat described how various studies using different methods developed precise knowledge of the possible risk of rubella at different stages of pregnancy. Research was then undertaken to develop an effective vaccine. Two major policy options emerged. The first was to attempt to eradicate the disease by vaccinating the entire population and maintaining its immune status; the second was to identify and immunise those at greatest risk to prevent them from developing the disease. The necessary investigations for such strategies are described in Lechat's review.

A different set of concerns – namely, policies on access to health services – were reviewed by Gulliford and Morgan.[13] The concept of access to health services is of major universal concern and is extremely complex. This review discussed some of the problems and measures required in order to assess such factors as availability of the service and its accessibility, accommodation, affordability and acceptability. Their study describes the types of questions patients should be asked about these five factors that will influence their use of services. The answers to these questions should be considered before any procedure is introduced into practice.

The effectiveness of a specific preventive policy was addressed in studies to determine whether the fluoridation of the water supply influences the development of dental caries[14] – an example of a pure epidemiological investigation with important implications for the provision of dental services. Other examples of apparently simple HSR investigations were those on the provision of food for hospital patients that were important in highlighting deficiencies in this area and in suggesting possible improvements.[15] As a result, the Department of Health now recognises that hospital food is an important part of patient care and, together with the Hospitals Caterers Association, has published practical guidance. Complaints about hospital food persist but the gross inadequacies in some hospitals, particularly in geriatric units, are now much less common.

The interaction of different methods of investigation and intervention is illustrated by the studies of methods for the prevention of coronary heart disease in North Karelia, Finland.[16] Initial studies showed that this part of Finland had one of the highest death rates from coronary heart disease in the world. Investigation of the habits, lifestyle and environment of the local population suggested a number of possible risk factors, including diet and smoking habits. Various methods were used to try to improve the situation: the fat content of meat products for sale was reduced; people were advised about their smoking habits and their cholesterol levels; individuals identified as having raised blood pressure were given appropriate advice and treatment. The health of this population improved dramatically. These experiments were a successful example of the need for cooperation between those concerned with public health in the widest context and those involved in the provision of health services.

Health Care Research and Health Policy Analysis

It is impossible to overstate the importance of good communication between HSR workers and health care policy-makers. Since the research worker is seldom responsible directly for health care planning or policy-making, it is essential that a satisfactory interchange of ideas occurs early in the formulation or resolution of policy issues.

Some authorities suggest that HSR and health care policy analysis are separate entities. Klarman[17] claimed that the time and programme scales of research and policy differ fundamentally. The objective of research is to describe the situation before and after the introduction of a health care programme with a description of the programme and, if possible, its effects. At the level of health care policy analysis, however, research by itself cannot always provide clear guidance on the setting of priorities. These will always involve other political or time factors.

Klarman sees research as describing the real world and testing hypotheses about how a given state came to be and policy analysis as listing and appraising alternative future outcomes. Both HSR workers and policy analysts must be able to deal with the uncertainty of outcomes or conclusions.

In spite of these differences, Klarman believed that the same individual may sometimes be able to perform both research and analysis as long as the worker or unit acknowledges clearly which activity is being undertaken at a particular time. The difficulty of communication between the policy-maker and the researcher, and the timescale involved, are crucial issues. It may be possible for the researcher to act both as researcher and policy analyst but it is a difficult role to fulfil effectively. The researcher may require more stringent data for arriving at decisions than the policy-maker who is constrained partly by political and time factors. The policy-maker may thus have to make decisions based on inconclusive or incomplete data.

More often and more satisfactorily, the researcher and policy-maker work separately while in communication. In this way, the researcher can be independent of those concerned with the formulation and implementation of policy decisions and the policy-maker can have a more objective view of the feasible options.

It must also be accepted that HSR does not stop once a policy has been agreed. The time interval between decisions on introducing a particular health care service and full-scale implementation, after pilot studies, is usually long enough for adequate research to be undertaken to evaluate its effectiveness and outcome and to make adjustments as necessary.

It is clear that such a role for HSR depends heavily on the type of organisation and network which links it to the decision-making centre of the health care system.

Three main streams of activity relate HSR to health care policy analysis.

1. Examining Policy Options
    In this application of HSR, an attempt is made to forecast the effects of implementing specific health care policies so that politicians and administrators can have as much information as possible on which to base their choice of available options. This may require action research on a small scale or purely theoretical modelling. Examples can be found in areas such as policy relating to immunisation programmes,[12] antenatal care,[18] obstetric care,[19] and care for the mentally ill.[20] Policy analysis must also show the assumptions and value judgements on which different policies are based.

2. Determination of selective factors influencing the distribution of existing programmes
    In this activity, HSR identifies factors such as demography, available manpower, available hospital or clinic resources, or economic characteristics that influence the use of facilities. Such research may be related to the overall regional resource allocation or the reallocation in single regions between capacity services. Typical examples of this in different areas are in the document by Katz et al.[21]

3.   Changes in health care practice, policy, law or administration in
        relation to defined disease phenomena
        As suggested previously, changes in the industrial, social or eco-
        nomic framework of a society may have serious implications for
        health care. Furthermore, discoveries about biomedical phenomena
        arising out of basic or clinical research can have value to a society
        only when these findings have some application in the health care
        system of that region. Thus, for example, HSR will be needed in
        the technical, administrative and legal formulation of programmes
        concerned with combating old and new bacteriological environ-
        mental or food hazards to health. Existing disease surveillance
        methods and registers can also be used within the ambit of
        HSR.[22, 23]

HSR is thus an essential tool of administrators and politicians responsible
for formulating and operating national or regional health care systems.

POLITICAL AND ADMINISTRATIVE FRAMEWORK

There are two models for engaging with HSR, as illustrated in Figure 1.1.
In Model A there are three players – the researcher, the policy-maker and
the provider, all of whom may interact. In most cases, using this model,
the researcher will be requested to provide the policy-maker with
scientific data on which to formulate a policy. The policy-maker will then
communicate this to the provider. In the more complex and more usual
Model B the policy analyst becomes a fourth player and there is full
interaction in identifying a research problem, providing a scientific basis
for various policy options and reaching a decision.
    The need for these complex inter-relationships can bedevil the
performance of the research work and the acceptance of results. Competent and valid research requires the freedom to explore and evaluate the
performance of providers and policy workers who may be constrained by
various time, financial and political considerations. Conflicts and misun-
derstandings can arise and create serious problems between and among
researchers, providers and policy workers. If, for example, a study of
services in an outpatient clinic revealed evidence of low productivity, the
clinicians concerned could deny the research team access on the assumption that high productivity must be good. This is of course not necessarily
the case and the researchers should help by examining the facts,
challenging the assumption and re-establishing access. Research evidence
of an unsatisfactory outcome from a particular policy decision may also

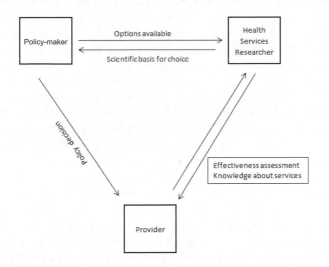

Model **A**

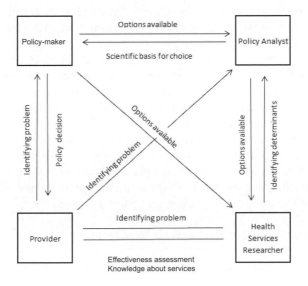

Model **B**

Figure 1.1   Models summarising the interaction between health service researchers and those concerned with making health policies and health service providers

create difficulties and may lead to political or administrative action to withdraw financial support from the research team.

An example of this was seen in the work of the Research Allocation Working Party (RAWP – see Chapter 6). This group produced a series of suggestions to improve the allocation of resources that were implemented for about ten years. The allocation formula devised was, however, attacked by other researchers, politicians and administrators who succeeded in having it modified in a number of ways. The original researchers were excluded from all discussions of the alternatives.

It was Mechanic who identified the vulnerability of this type of research as being caused partly by the absence of a clear constituency to promote it.[24] The study of conditions such as cancer or mental illness is usually supported by highly organised professional groups including clinicians, biochemists and psychologists. In addition, disease-based research often commands political and administrative support because of the emotional appeal associated with cure or care of the disease. HSR in contrast – being focused on services and prevention rather than on individual patients needing treatment – can be handicapped by unrealistic expectations and erratic changes in support of the research programmes by the funding agencies.

The HSR worker must be closely involved with health care policy-makers and providers while at the same time remaining free from undue influence and control to ensure the integrity of the research. Resolution of this paradox requires an appropriate administrative and political framework within which HSR can be contracted and performed. This framework must decide first on the best methods of organising HSR within the community's health services, second on appropriate funding, and third on the research agenda.

All decisions must relate to the way in which health care is itself organised within a particular society and to the general level and availability of other professional and academic resources or institutions. It is essential for all those involved in this process (see Figure 1.1) to agree at the outset on the outcomes to be achieved.

Organisation of Health Services Research

Whatever the method of organisation, a substantial governmental role will inevitably be part of the structure. In societies in which health care policy and health care services are provided directly from the public purse such an involvement needs no justification. But even when the health care system contains a substantial component of private medical and health care services, there will be need for government involvement – indeed, in such mixed health care systems Mechanic's argument[24] holds even more strongly when the influence of professional organisations and the competition for research funding will tend to deprive HSR of either constituencies or resources.

Because of the political nature of health care provision, government involvement is essential. Without it, it is inconceivable that valid HSR can occur or the results be used. The potential resistance to HSR by professional, health care or academic institutions requires an absolute commitment by government agencies to the research programme.

Models of Administration

Assuming a substantial role for government, there are several ways in which such administration can be organised.

Governmental models

Model A central government health services research units   The most obvious model is one in which the research organisation is directly incorporated into the health care policy and administration department of central government. In this case the HSR staff are direct employees of government and subject to conditions that apply to a central bureaucracy. Theoretically at least, such an organisation maximises the involvement of its staff in the policy analysis aspects and formulation of HSR. But equally this model might well minimise the freedom of action of research workers in their contacts with direct health care providers and create antagonism between researchers and providers. It might also run the risk of isolating research workers from their professional peers elsewhere in the scientific community. In a privately funded health care system the researchers could be associated with state control rather than policy formulation. This was the model used in the UK before 1967 and is described in this and the next chapter.

Model B regional government health services research units   Where the health care system has a strong regional administrative base it is clearly possible to develop HSR units within this administration. This type of organisation might be expected to have a closer interaction both with regional administration and the health care providers but could suffer as a result of its separation from the central policy-making apparatus. The research worker would be a government employee and freedom of action could, therefore, be curtailed to some extent by the conditions of employment. This model of organisation might also result in variations between regions in methods used and standards applied – useful perhaps for the purposes of comparison, but potentially harmful if the quality of research work is variable. This method of investigation was used in some US states including California.

Model C government subcontracted research organisations   This model is one in which the State's health care administration provides only administrative support to HSR units and finances the development selectively within other institutions. In this model, the units are developed outside the state agency while control is exercised through deferred accountability relationships between the unit directors and staff and the appropriate government department.

Unit staff can be employed either as civil servants or by the institutions in which the units are housed. In theory these institutions could be universities or other tertiary level institutions, hospitals or other health care establishments, professional organisations or private research foundations. The exact nature of the institution could be determined by the need for particular skills, the availability of an appropriate existing infrastructure or simply for regional convenience.

This model of organisation would have the maximum intellectual or academic freedom, helpful influence and contact with health care providers, and readily available peer professional support but would tend to lack involvement with policy analysis and decision-making. It is essentially the model now adopted in the UK.

Model D government financed independent health services research council   In this model, the central organisation is a separate council that administers and develops research units housed in other institutions. This may seem to be only a minor variant of Model C but the interposition of the research council (accountable to the government and accepting accountability from the research units themselves) may create additional difficulties. This model has been used to provide government funded biomedical research and is exemplified in the UK by the Medical Research Council.

This model maximises independence but minimises involvement with policy-makers or with the institutions of the health care system itself. It is appropriate to biomedical research where, as suggested, the questions are mainly those posed by the research workers. Where there is a need to consider health care problems closely related to the administrative or political structure of the state and its health care system, it has serious disadvantages.

Non-governmental models

It is possible to have HSR development pursued as a supplementary resource outside actual government control. The medical schools and departments or institutes of economics or social medicine may all contribute to the performance of research. The advantage of some extra-governmental direction of research relates to the need to encourage individually gifted research workers and the capacity to explore or innovate in terms of both study areas and methods using the enormous range of interdisciplinary knowledge and skills involved in HSR. In the US private foundations played a key role in the development of HSR. In the UK, independent bodies – notably the Nuffield Provincial Hospitals Trust and the King's Fund – were important players.

The Research Agenda

Directly related to the determination of organisation and funding is the question of who should specify the research priorities. A substantial proportion of the responsibility and funding for HSR should be the direct concern of the state health agency or department. Thus, by implication, this department should have a significant, although not absolute, voice in the specification of the research agenda. As indicated earlier, there is a serious administrative difficulty in attempting to give autonomy to research workers while at the same time ensuring that the research has relevance to clinical or bureaucratic decision-making. This can be resolved to some extent by having a form of administration that gives some financial independence to the research worker.

In his discussion of this problem, Klarman[17] attached most importance to maintaining the independence of the research worker, particularly as this related to the approaches, techniques or methods of research. This viewpoint assumes good personal but not necessarily over-formalised relationships between, for example, policy-makers and research workers. It can equally be argued, however, that it is necessary to formalise the link between bureaucrats, health service providers and HSR workers so that there is little dependence on individual personalities, a potential source of friction.

One compromise is to encourage good liaison between those who have to make the decisions, either centrally or regionally, and those who attempt to provide the solutions (HSR units). It is essential that the director and senior personnel of HSR programmes have personal contact with those who initially pose the problem. Equally, to accept Klarman's argument, these liaison groups should have no direct administrative function in managing the actual HSR programme.

METHODOLOGICAL FRAMEWORK

Developments in HSR must proceed in accordance with the nature of national health care services and within the political, economic and social framework of the state. The possible tasks of a HSR organisation are wide-ranging and can involve many scientific disciplines so that any general account of method would be inadequate. The main purpose of this section is to provide insight into the technical requirements of any national HSR programme.

HSR cannot easily be described by its individual academic components and this type of research does not develop in a vacuum. It must be assumed that in any political and bureaucratic state system, there are already some existing health care systems and educational institutions. In this context, it may be helpful to consider the skills that will be required in the development of a HSR programme and to look at the information and data systems involved.

Available Skills

An examination of the potential role of HSR suggests the need for individuals covering the following categories of knowledge: clinical medicine; laboratory medicine; epidemiology; statistical methods; computing; economics; social administration; sociology; anthropology; management services; and operations research (see Chapter 6).

Since the programmes will deal with health problems, health service personnel or institutions, it is clearly desirable to have at least one research worker with medical qualifications and experience in clinical, laboratory or investigative medicine. Almost all research programmes will involve epidemiological and statistical skills so that at least one person with these skills will again be a prerequisite of any programme. Any research agenda that seeks to explore behavioural or social aspects of illness or health care will need a social scientist, while studies of resource allocation or distribution will require an economist. Many studies will involve large amounts of data analysis and this can only be achieved by the use of computing techniques. Statistical skills will be involved and advice from computer staff, such as system analysts and programmers, will also be essential. In addition to these graduate skills, the research programme will call for support from secretarial, survey, data handling and library personnel.

Information and Intelligence Base

A HSR programme will usually develop within an existing bureaucracy and health care system and this implies the existence of an information and intelligence network already in use by the administration. This will vary in its completeness and complexity. At one level it may consist of a simple budgetary accounting mechanism for health care; at another it may be an extensive set of registers giving measures of mortality, morbidity, use of services and economic performance. Since this network can be a fundamental source of research data it is desirable to specify some essential components and to suggest that the establishment or extension of an ongoing intelligence system of this sort may well be the primary task of the research programme. This task once again demonstrates the need to involve governments in any health policy analysis and decision-making.

Data systems must be accurate so that researchers can have confidence in their use for analysing needs or options. The HSR worker should be involved in the establishment of such systems, if they do not already exist, or in their development, validation and use so that their full potential can be realised.

Possible Registers

Demographic data
Almost all countries register the births, marriages and deaths of their citizens by place of residence. This, with results of periodic censuses and estimates of migration, gives population estimates to provide measures of need for certain medical services. More information can be obtained by supplementing this with ad hoc additions to the registration form. Periodic national or sample surveys can also be used to determine living and economic conditions or the composition of households.

Economic and employment data
Most national governments record data relating to economic output or input. These include employment data, apparent food consumption, import or sales of tobacco and alcohol, chemical products imported or manufactured and details of expenditure within the health care sector and other parts of the economy. Such data are also an invaluable source of information about the use of or need for health care facilities as well as indicating some emerging or declining health hazards.

Mortality data
Every state records the cause of death of its citizens. These data may include occupational status as well as residence at the time of death and constitute one of the most important time series for all HSR. Large numbers of studies have used this kind of database, particularly when related to other population or economic trends.

Health service utilisation
Apart from financial data relating to expenditure or cost in the health care system, there are details of the reasons for admission to hospital or contact with a clinic. Many hospitals maintain their own record systems that give some idea of the use of health resources and recorded reasons for admission. Even at this level, useful information can be obtained by appropriate analysis and this will necessitate the skills associated with the HSR team.

Disease registries
Cancer registries exist and provide important additional data about illness. These registers have been used extensively as, at least, part of the database for HSR. Ad hoc studies can provide further information. Registries have been and continue to be developed for many other diseases including coronary heart disease, congenital malformations and stroke.

Ad Hoc Studies

In addition to the routinely collected data as described above, there is frequently a need to obtain further information by means of ad hoc studies in order to answer the questions posed to the HSR team. Such studies can be classified by the existence of factors determined by the time frame of collection, the type of method applied and the purpose of the study. The time frame is either *prospective* or *retrospective*. The method can be classified as *descriptive, analytical, comparative* or *experimental* although these terms are not mutually exclusive. The purpose of the study can be either: *basic* – for example, the development of methods to measure experimental clinical effectiveness, economic costs/benefits, provider and user satisfaction; *developmental* – for example, a community mental health programme; or *application-orientated* – for example, a primary health care system. This then gives rise to the following five types of enquiry.

1. Client/population surveys
    These can investigate many aspects of health care using interviews
    that may be self-administered or administered by a researcher. The
    survey is probably the single most important device for gathering
    information and has been used extensively to examine the use of
    services by clients, client or patient attitudes, symptom or illness
    occurrence and objective psychological or pathological changes,
    such as raised blood pressure or reduced lung function. In some
    cases, where there is a need to study a population over a length of
    time, longitudinal surveys may be necessary.

2. Surveys of providers or health service manpower registers
    Here the group interviewed are health care professionals. Surveys
    may be conducted merely to ascertain numbers, type or site of
    practice but they may also explore attitudes to patients, the work
    environment and work practices.

3. Technological assessment: need or performance
    Performance measurements or assessments of new or old tech-
    nology require comparative studies. In many cases the form of
    study requires identification of outcome and this may be immensely
    complicated. In more simple cases, such as assessment of drugs or
    antisera, the usual model adopted is the comparative clinical trial.

4. Cost-benefit/cost-effectiveness studies
    These studies attempt to determine the clinical or social effect-
    iveness or benefit of health care services in relation to economic
    parameters. Both cost and value may be expressed in cash or
    resource terms. These studies require various types of data input,
    some collected specifically for the model to which data are fitted,
    some cases involving the use of econometric models.

5. Theoretical modelling or simulation studies
    Some HSR studies may concern themselves solely with theoretical
    model building of the health care system. This has included
    theoretical models of institutions (operating theatres, outpatient
    clinics), manpower turnover and need, or total resource allocation.
    Usually data are collected from both ad hoc and routine sources and
    the model expresses the causal relationships inside the system being
    studied. Thus studies may be used in particular to forecast changes
    from alteration of or addition to policy decisions. However, the use
    of modelling or simulation studies to undertake investigation of
    total health care systems, whether regional or national, poses a
    large number of problems in view of their difficulty, the number of
    assumptions they involve, the need for extremely costly computing

equipment, and the highly skilled programming and systems analysis manpower required. In fact such national vast simulation-operational systems studies have so far contributed little to decision-making. The same caution may also apply to cost-benefit studies.

This list is not exhaustive but the range of methods once again reinforces the need for a considerable number of skills in the HSR programme. This need for a broad spectrum of human knowledge creates problems with data collection, analysis, interpretation and the communication of study outcomes.

Problems Associated with Health Services Research Methods

Apart from the usual technical problems of all experimental research such as the limitations of inductive reasoning, the need for reproducibility of results and estimates of error, HSR faces some special problems related to the context in which it is carried out. These can be summarised in four main categories: time constraints; comprehension of results; ethical and political constraints; and difficulties in communicating outcome.

Time constraints

Many of the processes which HSR studies use have a long and variable history. The processes may be very complicated and changeable. Indeed the very activity of studying a process involving humans, such as consultation by a health professional, may induce further changes in the process itself. Efforts to make short studies of long processes – for example, the development of cancer caused by industrial agents – seriously inhibits the acquisition or use of relevant knowledge. Furthermore the study of a complex process is difficult to formulate at the beginning of the study and the initial data acquired in a study may necessitate a change in the study protocol if it is to be relevant.

These problems occur much less frequently in biomedical research and this is apparent in the way in which such studies are assessed or financed. The HSR worker frequently has to contend with his or her research contractor, say a policy-maker, who needs results quickly in order to decide on a course of action. It is difficult then for the research worker to give a scientifically satisfactory solution which accords to the biomedical model and this limitation needs to be understood by all parties at the outset and a satisfactory compromise agreed.

Comprehension of results

There is a multidisciplinary output from many HSR projects. A cost-effectiveness study, for example, will contain biomedical information about effectiveness as well as economic information and assumptions. It is necessary, therefore, for research workers to be able to understand the logic of scientific disciplines different from their own. This in turn implies a need for senior multidisciplinary team members if worthwhile research is to be accomplished and adequate communication achieved.

Ethical and political constraints

The involvement of policy-makers or health care providers in posing problems to the HSR unit is essential. The outcome of such research may be required as part of a programme of health care service usage. This means that the research output has to be judged, in part at least, in terms of its utility in this respect. Here the research worker must meet constraints associated with ethical or political issues that will lie outside the purely scientific questions. At one level these cannot influence the scientific content but at another they cannot be ignored if the results of HSR are to be effective or put into practice.

Difficulties in communicating outcome

There is also a need to present scientifically based HSR, which may cover several distinct disciplines, in an understandable way to those who can use the results. In many instances the output of HSR is not adequately or properly implemented by clinicians or administrators.[25] This may be a result of a lack of the organisation essential for taking advantage of HSR, or because policy-makers and clinicians/providers of service are often unwilling to accept scientifically based results, preferring to rely on their own experience. Those involved in undertaking such research, therefore, must have good communication as well as research skills. The exposition of HSR must be communicated simply and without jargon in order to secure a commitment to the results.

CONCLUSION

Despite these constraints, HSR has come a long way in the last 50 years. In a rapidly changing world with many social, medical, environmental and cultural challenges, it is being increasingly recognised that clinical and curative approaches to medicine are not enough. HSR must underpin the workings of any successful modern health service. Its concerns with the quality, equity and effectiveness of health care make it ever more relevant in the twenty-first century.

REFERENCES

1   Global Advisory Committee on Medical Research (1983). *WHO Chronicle*, **37**(1), 4–5.
2   Flook, E.E. and Sanazaro, P.J. (eds) (1973). *Health Services Research and R&D in Perspective*. University of Michigan: Health Administration Press.
3   Academy of Medical Sciences (2005). *Strengthening Health Services Research*, 6 September.
4   Institute of Medicine: Division of Health Care Services (1979). *Health Services Research: a Report of a Study*. Washington, DC: Academy of Sciences.
5   Anderson, O.W. (1966). Influence of social and economic research on public policy in the health field: a review. *Milbank Memorial Fund Quarterly*, **44**, July Part 2, 11–48.
6   Sydenstricker, E. (1974). Hagerstown morbidity studies. Public Health Reports, 1926. In: Kasius R.V. (ed.), *The Challenge of Facts: Selected Public Health Papers of Edgar Sydenstricker*. New York: Milbank Memorial Fund.
7   White, K.L. (2007). Health services research and epidemiology. In: Holland, W.W., Olsen, J. and Florey, C. du V. (eds), *The Development of Modern Epidemiology*. Oxford: Oxford University Press, pp. 183–96.
8   McCarthy, T. and White, K.L. (2000). Origins of health services research. *Health Services Research*, **35**, 375–87.
9   Eisenberg, J.M. (1998). Health services research in a market-oriented health care system. *Health Affairs*, **17**, 98–108.
10 CIBA Foundation (1975). *Health and Industrial Growth*. Symposium 32 (new series). Amsterdam: Associated Scientific Publishers.
11 Holland, W.W., Bennett, A.E., Cameron, I.R., *et al.* (1979). Health effects of particulate pollution: re-appraising the evidence. *American Journal of Epidemiology*, **110**, 525–659.
12 Lechat, M.F. (1978). Causation and control with special reference to rubella. In: Holland, W.W. and Karhausen, L. (eds), *Health Care and Epidemiology*. London: Henry Kempton, pp. 228–42.
13 Gulliford, M. and Morgan, M. (eds) (2003). *Access to Health Services*. London and New York: Routledge, Taylor and Francis.
14 Ast, D.B. and Schlesinger, E.R. (1956). The conclusion of a ten-year study of water fluoridation. *American Journal of Public Health*, **46**, 265–71.
15 Platt, B.S., Eddy, T.P. and Pellett, P.L. (1963). Food in Hospitals: a Study of Feeding Arrangements and the Nutritional Value of Meals in Hospitals. London: Oxford University Press.
16 Puska, P., Tuomilehto, T., Salonen, J., *et al.* (1979). Changes in coronary risk factors during comprehensive five-year community programme to control cardiovascular diseases (North Karelia Project). *British Medical Journal*, **2**, 1173–83.

17 Klarman, H.E. (1980). Observations on health services research and health policy analysis. *Milbank Memorial Fund Quarterly*, **58**, 201–16.

18 Rumeau-Rouquette, C., Breart, G., Du Mazamburn, E., Crost, M., Arkhipoff, J. and Hermequinn, J.F. (1979). *Naitre en France. Enquetes nationales sur la grossesse et accouchement (1972–1976)*. Paris: Inserm.

19 Lazar, P., Servent, B., Dreyfus, J., Guegen, S. and Papiernik, E. (1979). Comparison of two successive policies of cervical cerclage for the prevention of pre-term birth. *European Journal of Obstetrics, Gynaecology and Reproductive Biology*, **9**, 307–12.

20 Ciompi, L., Agne, C. and Dawalder, J.P. (1978). Ein Forschungsprogram zur Rehabilitation psychisch Kranker: 2. Uberschnittsuntersuchung chronisher Spitalpatienten in einem modernen psychiatrischen Sektor. *Nervenarzt*, **49**, 322–8.

21 Katz, S., Ford, A.B., Downs, T.D., *et al.* (1972). *Effects of Continued Care: a Study of Chronic Illness in the Home*. Washington, DC: US Department of Health, Education and Welfare, Health Services and Mental Administration, National Center for Health Services Research and Development, DHEW public. No. (HSM) 73-3010.

22 Doll, R., Payne, P. and Waterhouse, J. (eds) (1966). *Cancer Incidence in Five Continents. Volume 1*. Berlin: Springer Verlag.

23 Langmuir, A.D., Henderson, D.A., Foege, W.H., *et al.* (1976). Symposium on methods of surveillance in planning for health. *International Journal of Epidemiology*, **5**, 13–91.

24 Mechanic, D. (1978). Prospects and problems in health services research. *Milbank Memorial Fund Quarterly*, **56**, 127–38.

25 Lewis, C.E. (1977). Health services research and innovation in health care delivery: does research make a difference? *New England Journal of Medicine*, **297**, 423–7.

2. Health services research in the United States

INTRODUCTION

The focus on HSR in the US – which developed earlier there than in the UK and before the Second World War – was largely with the distribution and utilisation of health services within the insurance system since there is no national health service. HSR was initially concentrated on the development of the basic disciplines, particularly sociology, the organisation of medical services and organisational structures, as well as the financing mechanisms for research.

HSR was also undertaken immediately after the Second World War in a limited number of organisations, such as the Veteran's Administration, the New York Department of Health and the Kaiser Permanente Health Foundation. The emphases for this research were on equity of access, moderation of costs and assurance of quality. HSR emerged as a distinctive activity in 1969 as part of the programme of the National Center for Health Services Research and Development. The programme was focused on improvement in the organisation, delivery and financing of health care through the introduction and testing in real community situations of carefully designed innovations in specific aspects of health care delivery. Among these areas of research which will be considered here were health manpower, health care facilities, organisation and administration of health services, evaluation, methods of financing health care, social behavioural aspects of health care, nursing, dental health, and health care technology. This chapter ends with a comparison of HSR in the US and the UK.

MANPOWER

This was one of the earliest areas in which HSR played a role in the US. In the early years, the main concern was with studies to determine the extent to which less qualified persons were practising in place of a physician. Anderson describes a study undertaken in Chicago in 1908 in collaboration with Hull House, on a birth record survey of midwifery in Chicago. A second study in Chicago, in 1930, showed that almost half the 40 000 birth-related deaths in Chicago were registered by midwives rather than by doctors.[1–3]

The most important report on medical education in the US is probably the Flexner Report which concerned the quality of medical education.[4] This report had an enormous impact on the type, quality and functions of doctors in the US. It was followed, in 1932, by reports of the Committee on the Costs of Medical Care and the use of non-medical personnel.[5]

During the 1940s Mountain and colleagues carried out further studies on the location and movement of physicians.[6] There were also a number of studies on surgical workloads and the shortage of primary care physicians.[7, 8] These basic studies were followed by other investigations of the work done by different types of practitioners, such as obstetricians, and studies were also undertaken of licensing and certification requirements.

HEALTH CARE FACILITIES

From 1909 the American Medical Association began to focus on information about the character and distribution of hospital facilities. By the mid 1930s, this strand of research had become much more systematic. It was taken over by the US Public Health Service and was part of the census of American business. The data produced were used by Mountain and colleagues in the study referred to above.[6] The American Hospital Association established a commission on hospital care and there followed a series of different studies measuring hospital capacity that were used in the context of the Hill Burton Hospital Building Programme after the Second World War. Studies of hospital costs and production of services were also started.[9, 10]

ORGANISATION AND ADMINISTRATION OF HEALTH SERVICES

Various studies were undertaken of public programmes of state agencies, and of the operation of units of local government, such as cities and counties, in the delivery of public health services. These studies were conducted mainly under the direction of Dr Joseph Mountain (see above) and were supplemented by the national health surveys already being undertaken during the 1930s – see for example, Mountain and Flook's study of the distribution of health services in the structure of state government.[11]

The private sector was examined far less stringently. Until 1950, the primary subject of inquiry was the organisation of medical care as a group medical practice. The Commission on Chronic Illness was established in 1949 and this, together with a variety of other organisations, such as the American Hospital Association, the American Medical Association and the American Public Health Association, undertook a number of descriptive studies of the medical care received within the private sector – see for example, the studies on homecare,[12] family practice[13] and paediatrics.[14]

EVALUATION AND QUALITY OF HEALTH SERVICES

The evaluation of health services only really began in the US in the late 1930s. This could be divided into: the evaluation of public health programmes; the development and application of methods for evaluating quality; and the evaluation of specific aspects of medical care, using social science and economic techniques.

Evaluation of Public Health Programmes

An important early example of this type of largely descriptive evaluation was Sydenstricker's study on the measurement of public health work which attempted to evaluate the work of the various state or county health departments.[15] This followed the work of Palmer.[16] More specific aspects of the work of health departments concentrated mainly on children and school health services.[17–19]

Evaluation of Quality of Medical Care

This type of work was started by Cabot in 1912 and extended by Codman two years later.[20, 21] The next major contribution in this area was the classic 1933 report by Lee and Jones on the fundamentals of good medical care.[22] Statistical methods began to be applied by Ciocco, in studying the quality of care in a group practice, and by Lembcke, in comparing rates with specific operations among hospital service areas.[23, 24] Lembcke was the first to develop explicit criteria and standards for diagnosis, treatment, hospital admission and length of stay on the basis of medical audit. He demonstrated the scientific and professional feasibility of this approach in major female pelvic surgery and it was adopted by a variety of different hospital associations, particularly in Michigan.

These studies demonstrated the importance of completeness, reliability, accuracy and validity of information contained in the clinical record if it was to be used for evaluating the quality of medical care. The limitations of having to use past medical records because of their neglect of assessment of reliability, validity and completeness were demonstrated in a number of other studies and thus had serious shortcomings.[25,26] The question of how to evaluate medical care and the necessary criteria for doing so was taken further by Eisele and colleagues[27] who demonstrated how accurate, objective data can be used to evaluate the quality of care more effectively than the use of judgement alone.

Research in the assessment of physician performance was given impetus by Peterson and colleagues who conducted and reported a study of general practice in North Carolina, using the technique of direct observation to determine if physicians performed in accordance with standards taught in medical school.[28] This study was important in demonstrating that the method of direct observation can be applied in the actual practice setting. It was also the first study to analyse the association of observed performance with personal, professional and educational background.

The critical incident technique (examining specific events in the care of a disease) was used to define the categories of physician performance reported to have beneficial or detrimental effects on patients.[29] It was Donabedian, however, who put forward the concepts of structure, process and outcome in his definitive summary and analysis of research of the quality of care.[30] In their subsequent study, Brook and Stevenson refined Donadebian's techniques and replicated both his methods and his findings.[31] Bunker[32] and Lewis[33] analysed the wide variation in rates of operation between countries and within states. Coronary care units were analysed with respect to end results, cost and productivity,[34] while Fanshel and Bush proposed a conceptual model for determining outcomes objectively.[35] Roemer and colleagues proposed an index of hospital quality based on a variety of criteria such as organisation, finance and measure of quality of medical care.[36] Huntley and colleagues studied the quality of care in the outpatient clinic,[37] while Shapiro and colleagues compared prematurity and perinatal mortality under the Health Insurance Plan of Greater New York, and in a sample of the general population.[38,39] Garland undertook some important work on observer variability in these types of study.[40]

Various different techniques were developed in the 1950s and 1960s to investigate the quality of medical care. The systems approach was examined,[41,42] and a variety of sociological methods developed.[43] Reader and his colleagues undertook a ten-year sociological study of the comprehensive medical care teaching programme at one hospital.[44] Economists, most notably Klarman and Andersen, undertook a variety of cost–benefit studies.[45,46] Quasi-experimental designs were used to determine differences in the effectiveness of organised programmes in achieving specified objectives. Goodrich and associates compared the effects on elderly welfare recipients of an organised programme of comprehensive medical care with those of the usual fragmented care, and found no difference in mortality or morbidity.[47] Robertson and colleagues conducted a controlled trial which demonstrated the effectiveness of a comprehensive health care programme in reducing the costs of illness.[48] Katz and colleagues undertook a controlled study of outpatient treatment in rheumatoid arthritis.[49]

Utilisation of health services was studied as early as 1927 by Sydenstricker in a landmark study of morbidity in the population laboratory of Hagerstown with the objective of defining the incidence of illness in the general population of a small city.[50] This was the first recorded study to relate services received by those who were ill and by diagnosis in a defined population. Collins reported the frequency of specific types of health services received by 9000 families, canvassed periodically between 1928 and 1931.[51-3] These surveys recorded health examinations, immunisation and related procedures, and doctors' calls.

After 1950, studies on different aspects of hospital utilisation began to increase, such as those on prolonged hospital stay[54] and the use of outpatient facilities.[55] Other examples of such studies are those by Densen and colleagues[56] and Roemer[57] which were concerned with the relationship between utilisation and prepaid medical care, and by Shain and Roemer[58] which related to costs in relation to the number of beds available. These studies of group practice and medical organisations continued throughout the 1960s. A number of authors examined the length of inpatient stay in various departments of the hospital in relation to bed supply, physician supply and costs.

Many of these studies related to specific occupational groups but they also extended their scope to look at particular groups, such as those patients in long-stay hospitals. Studies by Anderson and colleagues were probably the most systematic and widespread investigations of this type. They were concerned not only with utilisation of hospital services but also provided the most comprehensive information on the use of health services by different economic groups, were based on nationwide surveys and included investigations of cost.[59-61] These studies are a good example of perhaps the most systematic studies continued over many years of hospital utilisation by the Health Services Administration Center in Chicago.

Other studies in the 1960s and 1970s were undertaken by eminent investigators such as Sheps and colleagues, Last and White, and Bice and colleagues, who studied specific aspects of medical care utilisation, such as families in relationship to their normal doctors, the medical care provided in primary care and, most interestingly, the relationship of utilisation to poverty.[62-4] A useful comprehensive list of all publications on this subject was produced in 1972.[65]

ECONOMICS, COSTS AND FINANCING OF HEALTH CARE

The Committee on the Costs of Medical Care was the first group to address the problems of economics, costs and financing of health care. This was established in the 1930s and produced a large number of different reports. Reed, for example, examined the ability to pay for medical care.[66] Falk – a prominent investigator in this field whose interest in the costs of medical care continued for many years – published a report with colleagues in 1933 on the economic aspects of prevention and care of illness.[67] Studies, financed by the Milbank Memorial Fund, by Davis and Rosen on the crisis in hospital finance[68] and by Falk on health insurance,[69] are of particular importance in this context.

This interest with costs and health insurance continued for many years and Anderson was one of the most prominent workers to become involved. His paper on family medical costs and voluntary health insurance is illustrative of the studies on health insurance in the US.[70] Many reports were published over the years on this subject, including detailed studies of hospital and medical economics by McNerney, a future president of the American Hospitals Association, and supported by the W.K. Kellogg Foundation.[71,72] Other prominent health economists, such as Klarman, Feldstein and Reiss, also became involved in this field. Chicago and the University of Michigan was a centre for this work.

SOCIAL BEHAVIOURAL ASPECTS OF HEALTH CARE

Social behavioural research in health care really began in the US with the sociology of rural areas. One of the first such investigations was

Duncan's study of social research on health published in 1946.[73] Otis
Duncan was a quantitative sociologist who helped to introduce path
analysis to sociology. His later work was concerned with socio-economic
status and social mobility.

One of the most influential sociologists to study aspects of health care
and the health care professions was Freidson with his study on the
profession of medicine.[74] He attempted to improve the understanding of
the nature and potential of medical sociology as well as the attitudes,
motivation, behaviour and values of the consumers of health care. Many
of Freidson's studies were concerned with social structure, lines of
authority, communication and perceptions. There were, of course, also
studies on sociocultural aspects of health care, as well as physician–
patient interactions and relationships, and these were well summarised in
1963 by Freeman and colleagues.[75] The second edition of their book,
published in 1972, gives a good account of subsequent studies on
sociocultural aspects of health care and on patient-provider communica-
tions.

NURSING

The contribution of nursing to HSR has of course been a source of
investigation by many since the days of Florence Nightingale in the
mid-nineteenth century. In the US, however, comprehensive study on
such aspects as training, utilisation of services, as well as the adequacy of
services provided by nurses began in 1912. This work was followed by
studies undertaken by the New York Academy of Medicine which pointed
out a variety of inadequacies of nursing services.[76, 77] In 1940 the US
Public Health Service published the results of a major study on nursing
manpower.[78] Other research covered aspects of quality and evaluation,
both in hospital and in the community and outpatients, as well as social
behavioural research and economics and financing.

DENTAL HEALTH SERVICES RESEARCH

Dental services have long been the subject of studies in the US and have
been concerned with organisation and administration as well as social
and behavioural aspects. The utilisation of dental services, their economics, costs and financing as well as studies on evaluation were listed
in detail by Flook and Sanazaro in 1973.[79] Pharmacy-related HSR is also
covered by these authors in the same report.

HEALTH CARE TECHNOLOGY

Investigations on health care technology, in terms of HSR, only began after the Second World War, and were largely concerned with the use of computers, for example, in the automation of medical diagnosis, screening for disease detection, clinical laboratories, patient monitoring, medical records and hospital information systems. The work was concentrated in a relatively small number of sites and research was done in collaboration with private industry. Some of the first publications on the subject were by Ledley and Lusted[80] and Lipkin and Hardy.[81]

The development of automated hospital information systems (HIS), perhaps more than any other segment of health care technology, was spearheaded by private industry. It had been expected that this could be widely used in hospitals but many difficulties arose and the expectation was never fully realised. In 1968 Barnett, one of the leading investigators in this field, presented a somewhat critical analysis of the use of computers in patient care.[82] He was concerned with the use of computers in diagnosis and the interaction of computers with physicians. Barnett warned of the need for concern with the use of machines in these activities rather than humans who were able to identify such subtle factors as behaviour or appearance which influence physician–patient encounters.

In the 1960s, Collen and colleagues from the Kaiser Permanente Health Foundation developed a series of studies on automated methods of multiphasic screening, including electrocardiographic diagnosis,[83] but perhaps the most fruitful area of investigation was on the automation of the measurement and collection of biological data.[84,85]

White provides an excellent historical description of the development of the application of epidemiology to HSR in the US as well as in some other countries.[86] He pays particular tribute to Jerry Morris from the Medical Research Council Social Medicine and Research Unit in London for his efforts in stimulating interest in the application of epidemiological methods to HSR in the US.[87] In 1952 Morris had attended a conference at the University of North Carolina on research requirements for health and medical care at which he delivered a keynote address that helped to establish 'a major research agenda, at what was the first new medical school in the US after the Second World War.' His scientific methods were far more developed for HSR than those in the US and many of these are detailed in the 1963 book by Freeman and colleagues mentioned above.[75] A common method of investigation which was developed particularly in the US was the family household survey. This was used by the Committee on the Costs of Medical Care, detailed above, as well as by a variety of studies in Hagerstown and elsewhere and also referenced earlier in this chapter.[50-52]

COMPARISON BETWEEN THE UNITED STATES AND THE UNITED KINGDOM

The preceding text has illustrated a variety of different investigations undertaken on HSR in the US, many of them before the Second World War, but also shows the rapid development of HSR immediately afterwards. The important difference between the US and UK has been the role of private foundations. In the UK, most HSR has been supported by the Department of Health, with some studies being funded by the Medical Research Council. The King's Fund and the Nuffield Provincial Hospitals Trust were also important in establishing some crucial initiatives and in providing an external method of asking certain questions, which might not be easily done by an official government body. But few major studies were undertaken solely by either of these bodies. The Nuffield Provincial Hospitals Trust in particular was concerned with developing critiques of the delivery of health services and provided important stimuli to investigations undertaken through funding and research carried out by the Department of Health or Medical Research Council supported investigations.

In contrast, in the US, major studies were initiated, not only by the US Public Health Service, as in its studies in Hagerstown, but also by many private foundations who played a historic role in pioneering the support of activities contributing to the advancement of HSR. Later organisations involved included the Carnegie Foundation, the Josiah Macy Jr Foundation, the Milbank Memorial Fund, the New York Foundation, the Rockefeller Foundation, the Julius Rosenwald Fund, the Russell Sage Foundation and the Twentieth Century Fund. These all contributed to the financing, for example, of the Committee on the Costs of Medical Care. The Commonwealth Fund, the W.K. Kellogg Foundation and the National Foundation for Infantile Paralysis financed work by the Commission for Hospital Care, while the Rockefeller Foundation and the Commonwealth Fund contributed to the Commission on Chronic Illness. These foundations were involved in studies on the natural history and control of specific disease, as well as the training and education of professional health personnel and the improvement of health facilities and services.

The Milbank Memorial Fund, founded in 1905, had the longest history of supporting programmes and activities in the field of HSR. Very similar to the Nuffield Provincial Hospitals Trust, it did not have a very large budget but its impact was substantial, mainly because of the wisdom of its directors in directing enquiries to specific key areas that required investigation. These included the organisation of local public health services in New York State, population projects such as demographic studies and evaluations of different methods of delivery of health services. The Milbank Memorial Fund was particularly important in that it developed a publication that provided a respected forum for the publication and dissemination of the results of HSR.

The Commonwealth Fund, a much larger and wealthier foundation, was concerned with the development of demonstration projects – for example, providing model child health services. These were considered important since they were carried out in collaboration with State Health Departments rather than as isolated ventures. Projects included the Homecare Plan for the Montefiore Hospital in New York, the programme of the Richmond Virginia Department of Public Health for the medical care of indigents, a study of the Health Insurance Plan of Greater New York of family experience with medical care, and a survey of chronic illness in Baltimore by the Commission on Chronic Illness.

The W.K. Kellogg Foundation, established in 1930, followed much the same pattern as the Commonwealth Fund. With different points of emphasis, it has probably made its greatest impact on the evolution of hospitals and related health facilities, developing its interest in Michigan's rural population.

The Rockefeller Foundation, with far greater financial assets than any of the above foundations, also covered a much wider range of activities in its programme. Its international efforts were worldwide in scope and included support of the agricultural sciences, arts and humanities, as well as biomedical, natural and environmental sciences and social sciences. It has placed much greater emphasis on basic research. Before 1925, the Rockefeller Foundation's contributions to HSR were an outgrowth of its programme for the control of such infectious diseases as hookworm, malaria and yellow fever. As a result of its concern with the control of disease, it recognised the need to train health personnel which led to support for Schools of Medicine, Public Health and Nursing, and direct aid to individuals to enable them to attend such institutions. In 1916, the Rockefeller Foundation subsidised the building and endowment of the School of Hygiene and Public Health at Johns Hopkins University, which was opened in 1918 and became the country's first complete training centre for public health officers. One of the most important influences of the Rockefeller Foundation on HSR was its support of fellowships for medical care studies and its support for individuals, such as Cecil Sheps, Leonard Rosenfeld and John Grant, as well as Alan Greg, Kerr White and Milton Terris, who have played an important role in the development of HSR in the US.

Professional organisations, such as the American Hospital Association and the American Medical Association, also played a role in the development of HSR in the US, particularly before and immediately after the Second World War. Federal government support before 1950 was provided through the direct conduct of studies and the provision of staff assistance to various committees and commissions undertaken by public health service staff – for example, the studies in Hagerstown and on the Committee on the Costs of Medical Care. McCarthy and White give an excellent description of the origins of HSR in the US, and Eisenberg has examined HSR in a market-oriented health care system.[88, 89]

Funding of HSR in the US is much more substantial than that in the UK although it is difficult to get precise figures of the amounts spent because of the different sources of funding. In 1992, the US spent about $28.7 billion on health research and development as a whole from federal sources only. The amounts of money spent on HSR in the UK are detailed in Chapter 5.[90]

The HSR study section of the US Bureau of Health Services undertook a review of HSR in the UK, by visiting the country. The six individuals in the team were all experts in the field and their objective was to see how HSR was progressing in the UK and what lessons could be learnt for the US. Their comprehensive report was published in 1968.[91] The study group noted that the concentrated focus has resulted in a research programme considerably narrower in scope than the range of such work being supported in the US. The review included scrutiny of the Medical Research Council units concerned with population research – for example, those led by Professor Morris and Professor Cochrane. The visiting party was particularly impressed by the series of studies that had an impact on health practice and also commented positively on the wider variety of efforts for computerisation related to hospital services than in the US. A major critical comment was that there was little theoretical input into HSR in the UK. It also noted the absence of multidisciplinary work except in one or two places, but commented favourably on the integration of research and application of findings in Scotland compared to the rest of the UK. There was felt to be a lack of administrative leadership in the health service.

Most HSR in the UK was seen as descriptive with three main purposes:

- to provide information for the generation of new hypotheses;
- to help in the development of planning;
- to evaluate current activities.

Most of the research, however, was felt to be merely a collection of facts with little apparent effort being made to generate and test new hypotheses. Studies of the outcome of hospital care, for example, replicated earlier findings that had not been used to develop new principles or theories, or even to suggest practical solutions to problems. In some instances, the reviewers stated that conclusions were actually exhortations to use more of the services that had been shown by the studies themselves to be ineffective! The basic impression of the visiting group was that the research was often too pragmatic, was not sufficiently critical of current activities and lacked a theoretical background.

Administrators appeared to show little interest in evaluating the effectiveness of their programmes. This may explain, at least in part, the minimal involvement of most British researchers in developing more sophisticated techniques. Only rarely were comparative studies done to compare the effectiveness of providing services for similar conditions using either hospital-specialist services or community services. In addition, output and outcome were not regularly differentiated. The group was also surprised at the lack of change in the NHS since its inception. Two areas considered particularly important and in urgent need of theoretical development were the functional inter-relationships of the components of a large-scale service-oriented organisation and goal-setting mechanisms in the social services. The NHS should provide an excellent social laboratory for such research.

A striking observation was the virtual absence of studies on quality of medical care and the apparently widely held belief that quality of physician care was not an appropriate subject for research. There was some measurement, indirectly, of general practitioner performance, such as hospital-based diagnostic services, but very little research on the workforce and how it should be trained. There was no evaluation of the need for postgraduate education or how it should be delivered, or the characteristics of successful practitioners or administrators.

There was a paucity of studies related to the role of health professionals, especially that of manager and coordinator, and the absence of research in defining the functions of primary physicians was unexpected. The lack of multidisciplinary research and of training was also considered strange.

For various reasons the survey team was unable to form a clear impression of the extent to which the results of HSR contributed to planning and to policy decisions within the NHS. The traditional method of establishing national policies was, and remains, to appoint commissions, committees and working parties that use research findings to a variable extent. These usually operate on the principle of consensus, putting forward a series of recommendations that reflect the balance between what is desirable and what is acceptable to those responsible for implementation. In addition, operational research, as it has been conceived and carried out, has had little opportunity to influence planning decisions because its limited focus has made generalisation difficult.

Another major reason for the difficulty in clarifying the relationship of HSR to national planning was the absence of a clearly defined planning mechanism within the Ministry of Health and across the NHS. Although the Ministry was legally responsible for planning, integration and coordination of facilities and manpower services into separate components in the service, the study group found little evidence that a definitive planning process had evolved.[i] They were also surprised that regionalisation in the NHS was limited to the hospital service and not to any other sectors so that the administrative boundaries differed for hospital, preventive and general practitioner services.

Support for HSR was seen to be much weaker than in the US. But there was an established interest in at least the Nuffield Provincial Hospitals Trust to finance HSR and to follow it up and disseminate results. The UK grant mechanisms were felt to be informal and not as well established as in the US. The visiting team considered the US research programme to be much more diverse. In the US, it could be considered as social–medical, because its dominant, theoretical frames of inquiry were derived largely from the social behavioural sciences. Operational research was much less extensive than in the UK and significant studies in hospital function were lacking. On the other hand, much more US research was done on exploring the many dimensions of the idea of quality of medical care and the study of patients' and professionals' perceptions of need for medical care. They considered that UK research techniques would have significant potential for the US with development of record linkage and development of health data banks, analysis of care needs for hospital patients, the investigation of architectural design and the development of appropriate record systems as in the Royal College of General Practitioners. They did not expect to find that the centralised administration of the NHS had not developed an effective planning mechanism.

---

[i] A planning unit had in fact recently been established in the Ministry of Health but the Ministry remained overtly non-directive.

CONCLUSION

This chapter outlines the major areas of concern for HSR within the US, the development of methods and the problems that existed. It also includes a review of the views of a group of US health service researchers and administrators of the discipline in the UK. This emphasises the major differences between the UK and the US. The latter has produced far more research on basic principles and methodology, as well as social aspects. The US researchers also criticised the absence of application of some of the findings in the UK and demonstrated their concern for the lack of any formal structure within the Ministry of Health on what problems should be investigated or what needs to be done. This criticism comes strangely from the US, where, in fact, there is far less concern with these issues. It demonstrates, however, a clear difference in approach – the US studies were largely stimulated by the concern of individuals or individual foundations rather than by the Federal government. It is noteworthy that although many of the studies examined were interesting and were applied in limited areas, none of them had resulted in any major change in the direction of health care policy, nor in dealing with the problems identified by the investigations. This was true for both the US and the UK.

Recognition should be given to the development of the methodology and underlying experience of HSR in the US before the 1970s. The above gives a comprehensive account of the types of studies done in the US from which much was learned – but it is noteworthy that these studies were often done in the underlying hope that they might help in the development of a universal health system. Thus many of the investigators labelled themselves as involved in social medicine. This hope of a universal health insurance or national health system disappeared rapidly in the more recent past and the studies undertaken were more limited – concerned with practical matters such as effectiveness, efficiency and economics. There was a fundamental belief that a market system was the answer to health service problems. Various models were developed – for example, prepaid medical practice, Kaiser Permanente, preferred provider organisations and a number of insurance models. Only the system of health care provided by the Veterans Administrations for ex-servicemen, however, resembled the UK NHS system.

The underlying motivation in the US was to reduce costs and improve quality of health care. The former rapidly became an illusion within a system based on 'fee-for-service', increase in technology and no real means to contain costs. The latter became an increasing focus in both studies and policy, especially as it could be used as a marketing tool for a particular health plan.

A few US health service researchers, such as White, cited earlier,[86, 87] extolled the work in the UK and tried to emphasise what lessons could be learned but had little effect on general attitudes or developments. In spite of valiant efforts by his disciples, such as Barbara Starfield,[92, 93] there was little if any development, for example, general practice and health service costs continued to rise. The US now spends considerably more on health services, as a proportion of GDP, than any other developed country and yet the outcome, in terms of population health, lags behind that of other countries. Strangely, UK governments, since about 2000, have advocated many of the models and methods used in the US for providing health care – and in particular have adopted market rhetoric and neglected the fundamental strength of the NHS in providing health care in relation to need rather than demand.

Major contributions to the assessment of the quality of health care were made by Donabedian[94-6] and Brook and colleagues.[97, 98] The RAND Corporation undertook an experimental study of health care costs, utilisation and outcomes between 1974 and 1982.[99-101] This assigned people randomly to different kinds of health insurance plans and thereby costs, and followed their behaviour. The experiment provided evidence that cost-sharing reduced inappropriate demands for health care but also reduced the delivery of needed care, particularly of the most deprived and children. Unfortunately this study, although well designed and continuing for a long period of time, was not large enough to give statistically significant results. It was criticised for not being representative of the US population and thus dismissed by those proponents of a 'free-enterprise' medical system.

Bunker and his colleagues published an attempt to measure the contribution of medical care to health and concluded that medical care contributes more than prevention to improvements in health.[102] Their research findings are of great interest, but rely on assumptions that can be challenged.

Eisenberg, the Administrator of the Agency for Health Care Policy and Research, gives an excellent description of the US system of support for HSR and the major areas of concern as quoted earlier.[89] This illustrates the wide variety of mechanisms for support of HSR in the US, as well as the types of problems tackled. It is impossible to give more than one or two exceptional examples, as I have done, of recent HSR. In view of the very much greater magnitude of available resources, the scale of the work undertaken is far greater than that in the UK – but, as in the past, the research is less related to provider-needs but more to the exploration of principles and methods – and far more research-driven.

REFERENCES

1   Anderson, O.W. (1966). Influence of social and economic research on public policy in the health field – a review. *Milbank Memorial Fund Quarterly*, **44**(3), Part 2, 11–48.
2   Midwives of Chicago (1908). *Journal of the American Medical Association*, **50**, 1346–50.
3   Abbott, G. (1915). The Midwife in Chicago. *American Journal of Sociology*, **20**, 684–99.
4   Flexner, A. (1910). *Medical Education in the United States and Canada: A Report to the Carnegie Foundation for the Advancement of Teaching*. New York: The Carnegie Foundation.
5   Reed, L.S. (1932). *Midwives, Chiropodists and Optometrists: their Place in Medical Care* (CCMC Report No. 15). Chicago: University of Chicago Press.
6   Mountain, J.W., Pennell, E.H. and Nicolay, V. (1942). Location and movement physicians – general observations. *Public Health Reports*, **57**, 1363–75.
7   Hughes, E.F.X., Fuchs, V.R., Jacoby, J.E., *et al.* (1972). Surgical workloads in community practice. *Surgery*, **71**, 315–27.
8   Schonfeld, H.K., Heston, J.F. and Falk, I.S. (1972). Numbers of physicians required for primary medical care. *New England Journal of Medicine*, **286**, 571–6.
9   Feldstein, M.S. (1965). Hospital cost variations and case-mix differences. *Medical Care*, **3**, 95–103.
10 Feldstein, P.J. (1961). *An Empirical Investigation of the Marginal Cost of Hospital Services*. Chicago: University of Chicago, Graduate School of Business, Graduate Program in Hospital Administration. Studies in Hospital Administration.
11 Mountain, J.W. and Flook, E. (1943). *Distribution of Health Services in the Structure of State Government*. Public Health Bulletin: No. 184, 3rd edn. Federal Security Agency, Public Health Service, Washington, DC: US Government Printing Office.
12 Littauer, D., Flance, I.J. and Wessen, A.F. (1961). *Home Care*. American Hospital Association, Hospital Monograph Series No. 9, Chicago.
13 Huntley, R.R. (1963). Epidemiology of family practice. *Journal of the American Medical Association*, **185**, 105–8.
14 Hessel, S.J. and Haggerty, R.J. (1968). General paediatrics: a study of practice in the mid-1960s. *Paediatrics*, **73**, 271–9.
15 Sydenstricker, E. (1926). *The Measurement of Public Health Work*. Annual Report of the Milbank Memorial Fund, pp. 1–35.
16 Palmer, G.T. (1925). *Health Survey of 86 Cities*. American Child Health Association, Research Division. New York: J.J. Little and Ives Company.

17 Palmer, G.T. (1934). *Physical Defects – the Pathway to Correction.* American Child Health Association, Research Division. New York: Lienz and Riecker Inc.

18 Nyswander, D.B. (1942). *Solving School Health Problems.* The Astoria Demonstration, sponsored by the Department of Health and the Board of Education of New York City. New York: Commonwealth Fund.

19 Yankhanen, C.S. (1952). Designs for evaluation needed in the school health field. *American Journal of Public Health*, **42**, 655–60.

20 Cabot, R.C. (1912). Diagnostic pitfalls identified during a study of 3000 autopsies. *Journal of the American Medical Association*, **59**, 2295–8.

21 Codman, E.A. (1914). The product of a hospital. *Gynaecology and Obstetrics*, **18**, 491–6.

22 Lee, R.I. and Jones, L.W. (1933). *The Fundamentals of Good Medical Care* (CCMC Report No. 22). Chicago: University of Chicago Press.

23 Ciocco, A., Hunt, H. and Altman, I. (1950). Statistics on clinical services to new patients in medical groups. *Public Health Reports*, **65**, 99–115.

24 Lembcke, P.A. (1952). Measuring the quality of medical care through vital statistics on hospital service areas. I Comparative study of appendectomy rates. *American Journal of Public Health*, **42**, 276–86.

25 Trussell, R.E., Morehead, M.A. and Ehrlich, J. (1962). *The Quantity, Quality and Costs of Medical and Hospital Care Secured to a Sample of Teamster Families in the New York Areas.* New York: Columbia University School of Public Health and Administrative Medicine.

26 Lerner, M. and Riedel, D.C. (1964). The Teamster study and the quality of medical care. *Inquiry*, **1**, 69–80.

27 Eisele, C.W., Slee, V.N. and Hoffman, R.G. (1956). Can the practice of internal medicine be evaluated? *Annals of Internal Medicine*, **44**, 144–61.

28 Peterson, O.L., Andrews, L.T., Spain, R.S., *et al.* (1956). An analytical study of North Carolina General Practice 1953–1954. *Journal of Medical Education*, **31**(12), Part 2.

29 Sanazaro, P.J. and Williamson, J.W. (1970). Physician performance and its effects on patients. A classification based on reports by internists, surgeons, paediatricians and obstetricians. *Medical Care*, **8**, 299–308.

30 Donabedian, A. (1966). Evaluating the quality of medical care. *Milbank Memorial Fund Quarterly*, **44**(3), Part 2, 166–203.

31 Brook, R.H. and Stevenson, R.L. (1970). Effectiveness of patient care in an emergency room. *New England Journal of Medicine*, **283**, 904–7.

32 Bunker, J.P. (1970). Surgical manpower, a comparison of operations and surgeons in the United States and in England and Wales. *New England Journal of Medicine*, **282**, 135–44.

33 Lewis, C.E. (1969). Variations in the incidence of surgery. *New England Journal of Medicine*, **281**, 881–4.

34 Bloom, B.S. and Peterson, O.L. (1973). End results, cost and productivity of coronary care units. *New England Journal of Medicine*, **288**, 72–8.

35 Fanshel, S. and Bush, J.W. (1970). A health-status index and its application to health service outcomes. *Operations Research*, **18**, 1021–66.

36 Roemer, M.I., Moustafa, A.T. and Hopkins, C.E. (1968). A proposed hospital quality index. Hospital death rates adjusted for case severity. *Health Services Research*, **3**, 96–118.

37 Huntley, R.R., Steinhauser, R., White, K.L., *et al.* (1961). The quality of medical care: techniques and investigations in the outpatient clinic. *Journal of Chronic Diseases*, **14**, 630–642.

38 The Committee for the Special Research Project in the Health Insurance Plan of Greater New York (1957). *Health and Medical Care in New York City*. Cambridge: Published for the Commonwealth Fund by Harvard University Press.

39 Shapiro, S., Weiner, L. and Densen, P.M. (1958). Comparison of prematurity and perinatal mortality in a general population and in the population of a prepaid group practice medical care plan. *American Journal of Public Health*, **48**, 170–187.

40 Garland, L.H. (1960). The problem of observer error. *Bulletin of the New York Academy of Medicine*, **36**, 570–584.

41 Horland, D. and McDowell, W.E. (1964). Measurement of patient care. I Approaches to the system's problem. *Nursing Research*, **12**, 172–4, 1963. II Hospital systems model. *Nursing Research*, **12**, 232–6, 1963. III A conceptual framework. *Nursing Research*, **13**, 4–7.

42 Maloney, M.C., Trussell, R.E. and Elinson, J. (1960). Physicians choose medical care: a sociometric approach to quality appraisal. *American Journal of Public Health*, **50**, 1678–86.

43 Pratt, L., Seligman, A. and Reader, G.G. (1957). Physicians views on the level of medical information among patients. *American Journal of Public Health*, **47**, 1277–83.

44 Reader, G.G. and Goss, M.E.W. (eds) (1967). *Comprehensive Medical Care and Teaching. A Report on the New York Hospital – Cornell Medical Center Program*. Ithaca: Cornell University Press.

45 Klarman, H.E. (1967). Present status of cost benefit analysis in the health field. *American Journal of Public Health*, **57**, 1948–54.

46 Andersen, S. (1964). Operations research in public health. *Public Health Reports*, **79**, 297–305.

47 Goodrich, C.H., Olendzki, M.C. and Reader, G.G. (1970). *Welfare Medical Care: An Experiment*. Cambridge: Harvard University Press.

48 Robertson, L.S., Kosa, J., Heagarty, M.C., *et al.* (1973). *Changing the Medical Care System: Report of an Experiment 1964–1968*. Springfield, VA: National Technical Information Service, US Department of Commerce, Report No. PB-220-941.

49 Katz, S., Vignos, P.J. Jr, Moskowitz, R., *et al.* (1968). Comprehensive outpatient care in rheumatoid arthritis: a controlled study. *Journal of the American Medical Association*, **206**, 1249–54.

50 Sydenstricker, E. (1927). The extent of medical and hospital service in a typical small city, Hagerstown. Morbidity Studies No. III. *Public Health Reports*, **42**, 121–31. Reprint 1134.

51 Collins, S.D. (1934). Frequency of health examinations in 9000 families. Based on nationwide periodic canvasses, 1928–1931. *Public Health Reports*, **49**, 321–56. Reprint 1618.

52   Collins, S.D. (1937). Frequency of immunising and related procedures in
     9000 surveyed families in 18 states (1928–31). *Milbank Memorial Fund
     Quarterly*, **15**(2), Part 2, 150–172.
53   Collins, S.D. (1940). Frequency and volume of doctors' calls among males
     and females, in 9000 families, based on nationwide periodic canvasses,
     1928–31. *Public Health Reports*, **55**, 1977–2000.
54   Rosenfeld, L.S., Goldman, F. and Kaprio, L.A. (1957). Reasons for pro-
     longed hospital care. *Journal of Chronic Diseases*, **6**, 141–52.
55   Odoroff, M.E. and Abbe, L.M. (1957). Use of general hospitals: factors in
     outpatient visits. *Public Health Reports*, **72**, 478–83.
56   Densen, P.M., Balamuth, E. and Shapiro, S. (1958). Prepaid medical care
     and hospital utilisation. American Hospital Association, Hospital Mono-
     graph Series No. 3 Chicago.
57   Roemer, M.I. (1958). The influence of physicians prepaid service on
     hospital utilisation. *Hospitals*, **32**, 48–52.
58   Shain, M. and Roemer, M.I. (1959). Hospital costs related to the supply of
     beds. *Modern Hospital*, **92**, 71–3 and 168.
59   Anderson, O.W. and Sheatsley, P.B. (1967). *Hospital Use: a Survey of
     Patient and Physician Decisions.* Chicago: University of Chicago, Center
     for Health Administration Studies, Research Series No. 24.
60   Anderson, O.W. (1963). The utilisation of health services. In: Freeman,
     H.E., Levine, S. and Reeder, L.G. (eds), *Handbook of Medical Sociology.*
     Englewood Cliffs, NJ: Prentice Hall.
61   Andersen, R. and Anderson, O.W. (1967). *A Decade of Health Services:
     Social Survey Trends in Use and Expenditure.* Chicago: University of
     Chicago Press.
62   Sheps, C.G., Sloss, J.H. and Cahill, E. (1964). Medical Care in Aluminium
     City. I Families and their 'regular doctors'. *Journal of Chronic Diseases*, **17**,
     815–26.
63   Last, J.M. and White, K.L. (1969). The content of medical care in primary
     practice. *Medical Care*, **7**, 41–8.
64   Bice, T.W., Eichhorn, R.L. and Fox, P.D. (1972). Socioeconomic status and
     use of physician services: a reconsideration. *Medical Care*, **10**, 261–71.
65   Adey, L.A. and Eichhorn, R.L. (1972). The utilisation of health services:
     Indices and correlates – a research bibliography 1972. Department of
     Health, Education and Welfare, Health Services and Mental Health Admin-
     istration. National Center for Health Services Research and Development.
     DHEW Publication Number (HSM) 73-3003.
66   Reed, L.S. (1933). *The Ability to Pay for Medical Care* (CCMC Report No.
     25). Chicago: University of Chicago Press.
67   Falk, L.S., Rosen, C.R. and Ring, M.D. (1933). *The Costs of Medical Care:
     the Economic Aspects of Prevention and Care of Illness* (CCMC Report No.
     27). Chicago: University of Chicago Press.
68   Davis, M.M. and Rosen, R.C. (1932). *The Crisis in Hospital Finance.*
     Chicago: University of Chicago Press.
69   Falk, I.S. (1936). *Security Against Sickness: a Study of Health Insurance.*
     Garden City, New York: Doubleday, Doran & Co.

70 Anderson, O.W. and Feldman, J.J. (1956). *Family Medical Costs and Voluntary Health Insurance: a Nationwide Survey.* New York: McGraw-Hill.

71 McNerney, W.J., *et al.* (1962). *Hospital and Medical Economics – a Study of Population Services, Cost, Methods of Payment and Controls.* Two volumes. Chicago: Hospital Research and Educational Trust. American Hospital Association.

72 University of Michigan, Bureau of Public Health Economics and Department of Economics (1964). *The Economics of Health and Medical Care: Proceeding of the Conference on the Economics of Health and Medical Care.* 10–12 May, 1962. Ann Arbor: University of Michigan.

73 Duncan, O.D. (1946). *Social Research on Health.* New York: Social Science Research Council.

74 Freidson, E. (1970). *Profession of Medicine: a Study of Applied Knowledge.* New York: Dodd, Mead and Co.

75 Freeman, H.E., Levine, S. and Reeder, L.G. (eds) (1963). *Handbook of Medical Sociology.* Englewood Cliffs, NJ: Prentice Hall. Second edition, 1972.

76 Nutting, M.A. and Dock, L.L. (1907). *History of Nursing.* Volume II. New York: GP Putman's and Sons.

77 Lewinski-Corwin, E.H. (1922). The hospital nursing situation. *American Journal of Nursing*, **22**, 603.

78 A national inventory of nurses (1940). *American Journal of Nursing*, **40**, 1246.

79 Flook, E.E. and Sanazaro, P.J. (eds) (1973). *Health Services Research and R&D in Perspective.* Ann Arbor, MI: Health Administration Press (pp. 49–55).

80 Ledley, R.S. and Lusted, L.B. (1959). Reasoning foundations of medical diagnosis. *Science*, **130**, 9–21.

81 Lipkin, M. and Handy, J.D. (1958). Mechanical correlation in differential diagnosis of haematologic diseases. *Journal of the American Medical Association*, **166**, 113–25.

82 Barnett, G.O. (1968). Computers in patient care. *New England Journal of Medicine*, **279**, 1321–7.

83 Collen, M.F., Ruben, L., Neyman, J., *et al.* (1964). Automated multiphasic screening and diagnosis. *American Journal of Public Health*, **54**, 741–50.

84 Hochberg, H.M., Calatayud, J.B., Weihrer, A.L., *et al.* (1967). Automatic electrocardiogram analysis in rapid mass screening. *Archives of Environmental Health*, **15**, 390–398.

85 Larson, B.G. (1965). Computer assisted data processing in laboratory medicine. In: Stacy, R.W. and Waxman, B.D. (eds), *Computers in Biomedical Research*, Volume 1. New York: Academic Press, pp. 353–76.

86 White, K.L. (2007). Health services research and epidemiology. In: Holland, W.W., Olsen, J. and Florey, C. du V. (eds), *The Development of Modern Epidemiology.* Oxford: Oxford University Press, pp. 182–96.

87 White, K.L. (2002). Jerry Morris and health services research in the USA. *International Journal of Epidemiology*, **31**, 690–693.

88 McCarthy, T. and White, K.L. (2000). Origins of health services research. *Health Services Research*, **35**, 375–87.

89 Eisenberg, J.M. (1998). Health services research in a market-oriented health care system. *Health Affairs*, **17**, 98–108.

90 Detels, R., Holland, W.W. and Tanaka, H. (1996). Organisational status of basic and applied research in public health. In: Hurrelman, K. and Laaser, V. (eds), *International Handbook of Public Health*. Westport, CT: Greenwood Press, pp. 19–51.

91 Bierman, P., *et al.* (1968). Health services research in Great Britain. *Milbank Memorial Fund Quarterly*, **46**, 9–102.

92 Starfield, B. (1990). *Primary Care. Balancing Health Needs, Services and Technology*. New York: Oxford University Press.

93 Starfield, B., Shi, L. and Macinko, J. (2005). Contribution of primary care to health systems and health. *Milbank Memorial Fund Quarterly*, **83**, 457–502.

94 Donabedian, A. (1980). *Explorations in Quality Assessment and Monitoring. Volume I. The Definition of Quality and Approaches to its Assessment*. Ann Arbor, MI: Health Administration Press.

95 Donabedian, A. (1982). *Explorations in Quality Assessment and Monitoring. Volume II. The Criteria and Standards of Quality*. Ann Arbor, MI: Health Administration Press.

96 Donabedian, A. (1985). *Explorations in Quality Assessment and Monitoring. Volume III. The Methods and Findings of Quality Assessment and Monitoring: an Illustrated Analysis*. Ann Arbor, MI: Health Administration Press.

97 Brook, R.H. and Appel, F.A. (1973). Quality of care assessment: choosing a method for peer review. *New England Journal of Medicine*, **288**, 1323–9.

98 Brook, R.H., McFlynn, E.A. and Shekelle, P.G. (2000). Defining and measuring quality of care: a perspective from US researchers. *International Journal of Quality Health Care*, **12**, 281–95.

99 Newhouse, J.P. (1993). *Free for All? Lessons from the RAND Health Insurance Experiment*. Cambridge, MA: Harvard University Press.

100 Manning, W.G., Newhouse, J.P., Duan, N., Keeler, E.B., Benjamin, B., Liebowitz, A., *et al.* (1988). *Health Insurance and the Demand for Medical Care. Evidence from a Randomized Experiment*. Report R-3476-HHS. Santa Monica, CA, RAND Corporation.

101 Brook, R.H., Ware, J.E., Rogers, W.H., Keeler, E.B., Davies, A.R., Sherbourne, C.A., *et al.* (1984). *The Effect of Co-insurance on the Health of Adults. Results*. R-3055-HHS. Santa Monica, CA, RAND Corporation, 1984.

102 Bunker, J.P., Frazier, H.S. and Mosteller, F. (1994). Improving health: measuring effects of medical care. *Milbank Quarterly*, **72**, 225–58.

3. Health and health services research in the United Kingdom: a historical review

HEALTH RESEARCH

Haldane

The introduction of scientific principles into Government decision-making really began with publication in 1918 of the Haldane Report and the Haldane Principle, a wide-ranging report on the machinery of Government after the First World War.[1] Richard Haldane, First Viscount Haldane, was one of the most influential figures in British politics in the early twentieth century, serving as War Minister from 1905 to 1912 and Lord Chancellor from 1912 to 1915. Although his report considered the relationship between Government and research in general, this was not its main purpose. The report was commissioned to enquire into the responsibilities of the various departments of the Central Executive of Government and to advise on the manner in which these could best be exercised. In preparing his report, he made various recommendations, stressing the fundamental need for research: 'Further provision is needed in the sphere of civil government for continuous acquisition of knowledge and the prosecution of research in order to furnish a proper basis for policy.'[2]

Haldane believed that research should play a key role in Government and the report included two main proposals. The first was that: 'In all departments, better provision should be made for enquiry, research and reflection before policy is defined and put into operation.'[3] Further, he stated: 'Many departments must retain under their own control, a distinctive organisation for the prosecution of specific forms of research.'[4] The second proposal on research was that: 'For some purposes, the necessary research and enquiry should be carried out or supervised by a Department of Government specifically charged with these duties, but working in the closest collaboration with the administrative departments concerned with its activities.'[3] He continued:

as regards the methods to be adopted for conducting enquiry and research in any branch of knowledge, so far as it is determined that the work should be carried out under the supervision of a general organisation, and not under that of an administrative department, we think that a form of organisation on the lines already laid down for Scientific and Industry research would prove most suitable.[5]

His model placed responsibility on Parliament in the hands of a Minister free from any serious pressure of administrative duties and immune from any suspicion of being biased by administrative considerations against the application of the results of research. Crucially, even for this kind of research for general use, Haldane did not propose that decisions about it should be taken at arm's length from Government. In fact, he proposed that these decisions should specifically be the responsibility of a Government Department, but not an administrative department with policy responsibility for the area of research in question. It is clear from this that the establishment of research councils to conduct research at arm's length from Government was a step beyond that recommended by Haldane. The Haldane Report also specifically examined in more detail the work of the predecessor to the Medical Research Council – that is, the Medical Research Committee which had been constituted under regulations from the National Insurance Act of 1911. This Act created the Medical Research Fund to which one penny was allocated for each person insured in the UK. Haldane noted that: 'The Minister responsible for health insurance never sought to control the work of the Committee or to suggest to them that they should follow one line of enquiry rather than another.'[6]

The work of the Medical Research Committee was certainly not at arm's length from Government. The first members of the Medical Research Committee, appointed in 1913, were made responsible for creating schemes of research and submitting them for scrutiny by a Minister. Approval had to be obtained before any money could be allocated. The Committee consisted of a member of the House of Lords, two members of the House of Commons as well as six scientific experts appointed by the Minister.[7] Haldane's evaluation of the Medical Research Committee was restricted to the years spanning the First World War. He stated that the Committee devoted almost all its energies to the investigation of problems arising out of war conditions which were then referred to the relevant administrative departments including the Admiralty, War Office, Air Ministry, Home Office and Ministry of Munitions. On the governance of research, Haldane concluded that:

It may therefore not be premature to anticipate that the distinctive character of the organisation of intelligence and research for general use; the proper scope of such an organisation and its potential relations with analogous organisations throughout the Empire could then support, or be maintained, by a Minister specifically appointed on the ground of his suitability to preside over a separate Department of Intelligence and Research, which would no longer act under a Committee of Privy Council and would take its place among the most important Departments of Government.[8]

Above all else, Haldane's vision was that research should be an integral part of the machinery of Government. His assessment of the Medical Research Committee as an entity devoted to problems arising out of the war conditions of that time illustrates a process whereby the Government of the day could refer its problems to the Committee[i] in a search for solutions.

Over the next 50 years or so, increasing levels of dissatisfaction were expressed about the nature of publicly funded research, especially in the area of health. The establishment of the NHS in 1948 introduced a Minister of Health with specific powers and responsibilities to pursue a programme of research to support its needs.[9] The Department of Health and Social Service (DHSS) started to commission substantial amounts of research in the late 1960s. Tensions developed on the demarcation of responsibilities between the Medical Research Council and Ministry research. Despite repeated attempts by the Department of Health to influence priority setting within the Medical Research Council, researchers were still largely engaged in knowledge-led investigations. In 1970, a White Paper on 'The Reorganisation of Central Government' recommended that at a high level in the policy-making system, there should be a small multidisciplinary Central Policy Review Staff (CPRS) in the Cabinet Office. This recommendation was implemented in 1971.[10] The CPRS was set up within the Cabinet Office and was intended to define Government strategy and develop it to take account of changing circumstances. The CPRS was also intended to provide a framework within which the Governments' policies as a whole might effectively be formulated. The first Director General of the CPRS was appointed in 1971 by the then Prime Minister, Edward Heath. He was Lord Victor Rothschild, Third Baron Rothschild, an eminent biologist who had also served as Chairman of both the Agricultural Research Council and Shell Research.

---

[i] Under the terms of the Ministry of Health Act 1919, the Medical Research Committee became the Medical Research Council, separate from the new Ministry of Health and with the same members and functions as its predecessor, but with the addition of a Royal Charter.

Under Rothschild's leadership, the CPRS studied fundamental aspects of Government policy, often crossing departmental boundaries, and drawing attention to the consequences of an action or inaction across the field of Government.

Addison

Overlapping all these concerns was the work of Christopher Addison, Chairman of the Reconstruction Committee, who discussed a variety of proposals and defended the principle of independent and undirected research. In 1919 Addison pointed out that the success of the general use approach could be illustrated by research into oxygen which had resulted in advances in aviation, mine rescue and pneumonia treatment. As such, the work had been of relevance to several different Government Departments. Addison was convinced that scientific freedom alone could produce the highest quality of work, and he worried that departmental direction would force scientists to concentrate too much on immediate needs and warned that ministerial control could jeopardise the rigour of scientific research with Ministers being tempted to interfere and to try to secure conclusions acceptable to them. Addison's plea was that scientists should be aloof from current demands of satisfying particular administrative needs.[11, 12] Haldane considered that Ministry research would largely be limited to surveys and statistics. Addison agreed that surveys and statistics were needed to illuminate policy but felt strongly that other 'free' research was needed and envisaged a degree of parity of expenditure between the two strands. Addison felt that much medical research could best be carried out by medical staff in close cooperation with the administrative side of the Ministry and by a body whose work would be less immediately directed towards the current administration of health matters. He concluded that Ministry research should respond to immediate needs whereas Medical Research Council research should be knowledge-driven and guard the freedom of the Council's researchers.

The first Secretary of the Medical Research Council was Sir Walter Morley Fletcher. He promoted an organisation that required to be shielded from external control and that also acted as a national body directing all medical research, including work funded through private donations. The proposals of Addison rather than those of Haldane were thus largely implemented. But relations between the two bodies – that is the Ministry and the Medical Research Council – became increasingly tense, particularly when a Departmental Cancer Committee was set up by the Ministry in 1923. In an attempt to resolve the situation, Fletcher and Sir George Newman, the Ministry's Chief Medical Officer, privately drew up a concordat that confirmed each body's profile. The new Ministry was to undertake investigation of scientific problems arising from its current administrative work with studies focusing on public health administration, applied knowledge or medical services.[12]

Because of inadequate external structures and internal capacity, government-led research was slow to gain momentum. The Ministry should have been well placed to combine health research with health care, but since the latter was regionally and socially fragmented, this did not happen. This situation improved slightly in 1946 when the National Health Service Act was passed[9] and the NHS offered a unified system for health care provision across the nation, open to everyone and free at the point of delivery. The 1946 Act explicitly put the Ministry of Health in charge of research into matters relating to causation, prevention and diagnosis of illness or mental deficiency – a broad remit, reminiscent of the original brief of the Medical Research Committee. But the vision was not matched by the means. Although clinical research began to expand in teaching hospitals, the Ministry's actual research programme remained confined to public health. Consequently, existing structures really prevailed until the 1960s when external pressure refuelled interest in the Ministry as a significant player in the research arena.

In the early 1960s there was a growing awareness of the need to undertake research but there were problems. The Ministry needed scientific knowledge about specialised subjects such as, for example, organ transplantation and population screening on which the Medical Research Council was unable to offer appropriate assistance. The Ministry thus stepped in to fill the gap by developing its own research capacity and research units.[13] At the same time, the Medical Research Council was undertaking public health studies alongside the Ministry and the research boundaries were becoming blurred. There were increasing problems in understanding what was immediate, applied or general work. The Chief Medical Officer perceived a lack of epidemiological focus in the Medical Research Council's work and matters were not helped because some in the scientific community still regarded work undertaken on behalf of the Ministry as being somehow second class. Wider society meanwhile began to exhibit signs of disenchantment with science that sometimes amounted to a veritable science counter-culture.

By the 1960s, the blurred relationship between the Medical Research Council and Ministry reflected a wider debate in Government about the best way to undertake publicly funded research. In 1964, a Government-commissioned enquiry into civil science, led by Sir Burke Trend, found

that endeavours had been weakened by a lack of clarity in the arrangements for coordinating the Government's scientific effort and apportion-
ing available resources between agencies on a rational basis.[14] The need
for more organised research gave rise to the idea that Government
departments should set the agenda for all publicly funded research in
their field. In the case of health research, this challenge to the Medical
Research Council had not been seriously considered since the reports of
Haldane and Addison when Addison had defended its independence.

In 1970 the idea of bringing the research councils under departmental
control was spelled out in an unpublished report on the Agricultural
Research Council led by Paul Osmond of the Civil Service Department.[15]
Shortly afterwards, the new Heath Government created the CPRS, as
mentioned above, and commissioned two reports.

Rothschild

The Rothschild Report examined the current department and research
council system, with the aim of determining the most effective arrangements for organising and supporting pure and applied scientific research
and postgraduate training. Rothschild believed that the individualistic
stance exemplified by the Medical Research Council was to blame for the
perceived unsatisfactory return in public investment in research. Effective
service for the Government, he argued, required a centralised and
needs-focused approach. Administrative departments did not require
scientific support, but applied research and development (R&D) projects
to achieve specific predetermined objectives. Rothschild's solution was a
radically new approach based on precise departmental commissions.
Applied R&D studies should be done on a customer-contractor basis –
the customers state what they want, the contractors do it if they can and
the customers pay. The report envisaged the Government departments as
the customers, or acting on behalf of the ultimate customers, and the
research bodies as the contractors. To empower the customers, the report
proposed that a large part of the funds previously allocated to the
research councils should be transferred to the departments. The research
councils would then have to win back this money by bidding for
departmental research contracts. At the same time they would not
normally be able to refuse departmental commissions. Knowledge-driven
research, a traditional domain of the councils, was to be financed by a
general research surcharge, factored into the price of commissioned
work. This system was expected to end the lingering scientific snobbery
dividing the 'haves' in the research councils and the 'have not's' in the
departments.[10]

Rothschild, therefore, negated the endorsement by both Haldane and Addison of research council independence and rejected the idea that departments and councils should occupy different positions on the basic–applied research spectrum.

Rothchild's third radical proposal called for the *National Research Agenda* to be taken out of the hands of scientists on the grounds that, however distinguished, intelligent and practical these experts might be, they could not be in as strong a position to decide on the needs and priorities of the nation as those responsible for ensuring that those needs and priorities are met. Rothschild, however, did not propose a department-led national strategy for health R&D. For him, priority-setting was a question of identifying immediate needs at local level and he, therefore, saw no need to track national R&D activity, arguing that such a general oversight would serve no useful purpose.

Dainton

The second report, published with the Green Paper, 'The Future of the Research Council System', scrutinised Osmond's proposal to bring research councils under ministerial control. It was led by a distinguished academic chemist, Sir Frederick Dainton, who concluded in favour of the councils' autonomous status. Echoing Addison's thoughts on the relationship between government and science, Dainton highlighted that independent research remained of great value in public decision-making. Departments need to be able to obtain help and independent advice free from considerations of administrative and political convenience.[16]

Dainton's Report emphasised the need to have unbiased expertise for the effective functioning of departments. The White Paper in July 1972 ensured the continuation of the independent research councils, but implemented most of Rothschild's proposals with the addition of a Supervisory Board of Research Councils recommended by Dainton.[17] This shift catapulted the DHSS into a national management and leadership position, assuming the final responsibility for defining the objectives of commissioned work although its research management experience was limited. The DHSS's R&D budget for 1972–1973 amounted to £13 million, including £9.3 million for current expenditure. Of the latter sum, only £0.7 million was earmarked for work done within the DHSS by its own researchers.

To oversee the DHSS's expanded R&D programme, the Government appointed a Chief Scientist who was supported by a small number of staff and several advisory bodies. Most notably, the Chief Scientist's Research Committee discussed suitable foundations for commissioning research, such as cost–benefit analysis and the analysis of future needs. At the same time, £5 million out of £20 million of public funds earmarked for the Medical Research Council was transferred to the DHSS – that is to say, approximately 25 per cent of the Medical Research Council's funding was to be spent on applied research. The DHSS was represented more strongly on the Board of the Medical Research Council as proposed by Rothschild. The reforms allowed for stronger central direction but were predictably unpopular with the scientific community. In particular, researchers protested that the Government had not analysed the supposed weaknesses of the previous system adequately.

Difficult Relationships

As the reforms were implemented, practical problems emerged. The research councils for example, found it difficult to raise funds for non-commissioned capacity building research because Government Departments were under no obligation to pay the new general research surcharge. Researchers were also disappointed that science had not gained more influence on policy-making. The subsequent relationship between the DHSS and the Medical Research Council revealed that departmental structures were insufficiently robust to allow authoritative decision-making within the new system. The DHSS not only needed to handle a greatly expanded budget but was also expected to allocate funding across all areas of health research. Given the limited capacity of the Chief Scientist's Office, this proved an overwhelming challenge. The problem was resolved by giving the Medical Research Council broad research contracts that effectively allowed the Council to continue its existing research programme. This move was pragmatic but ignored Rothschild's outspoken opposition to open-ended funding agreements. Medical Research Council researchers, meanwhile, continued to feel the reforms as a heavy administrative burden compounded by time-consuming obligations to act as expert advisors to the Government.[18]

This first radical restructuring of the system put customer and customer need theoretically at the centre, but the reality did not match the theory. Neither customers nor needs were adequately represented by the DHSS. The first Chief Scientist was Dr R.H.L. (Dick) Cohen. He was followed by Sir Douglas Black who considered that his remit in the post was advisory rather than executive. The disparity between the Government's aspirations for the new system and its practical shortcomings did not go unnoticed and led to a series of reports and subsequent reforms.[18-20] Maurice Kogan was asked to review the arrangements for DHSS research. He considered that the Office of the Chief Scientist

(OCS) was on the margins rather than at the centre of the organisation and, more seriously, that severe lack of scientific experience among staff was hampering the DHSS from devising its own projects. The internal structure of the DHSS was, therefore, remodelled. The Chief Scientist Research Committee was formed with more than ten research liaison groups (RLGs) intended to bring together departmental advisors, independent experts and DHSS staff. The new structure, however, was soon criticised as being over-ambitious and the RLGs did not actually have a definable research policy with sufficient overview of the fragmented customer-focused R&D activities normally under its control. This criticism from the Nuffield Provincial Hospitals Trust[15] was repeated in a review of civil service management.[21]

Part of the problem was that the reduction in civil service staffing and constraints on the size of the DHSS had an impact on its ability to manage the activities of the RLGs appropriately. Another difficulty with the groups was that their work was limited to a few very specialised priority areas such as mental deficiency and they neglected the major concerns of the DHSS, particularly the planning of general and acute health services. The RLGs met infrequently, had a high turnover of staff and did not command professional respect. The outcome of all the reforms, reports and debates was thus a hybrid of pre- and post-Rothschild models. There was no single decision-making body able to provide the necessary direction for research or find an appropriate balance between independent and commissioned knowledge-led and needs-based research. Other issues, such as the adequate range of scientific support and the effective linking of science and policy, also remained to be resolved.

The sort of problems that existed in the commissioning of research is exemplified in the studies undertaken at St Thomas' Hospital Medical School to determine whether the planned new District General Hospitals could perform their intended functions – that is, to produce a shift from inpatient to outpatient community care. The St Thomas' Unit put forward a number of proposals for these studies. At the initial meeting with the DHSS however, a senior departmental official raised the question of whether research that might question policy could be funded. The Chief Scientist and the researchers pointed out that the function of research was to question not endorse policy but the official remained firmly of the view that researchers could not question departmental policy. This produced an obstruction that took six months and ministerial involvement to resolve with an agreement that research could indeed evaluate and question policy.[22]

The changes in the structure of the research funding for health services then continued until the House of Lords, Science and Technology Committee reviewed the organisation of medical research in the UK. This is covered in detail in Chapter 7.

HEALTH SERVICES RESEARCH

Although the Ministry of Health had concerned itself with special studies – for example, confidential enquiries on maternal mortality – there remained a clear need for research capacity within the Ministry. The Ministry was required to be involved in studies to enable decisions to be made in planning and priority setting for the improvement of health care in contrast to the Medical Research Council which was largely concerned with basic and clinical research. The Ministry was also required to carry out research on personal social services for which there was no established research mechanism or research council. Any research on public health, one of the most important functions of the Ministry, was undertaken by the Public Health Laboratory Service (PHLS) under the aegis of the Medical Research Council.

The National Health Service Act of 1946 contained a clause which stated that:[9]

> without prejudice to the general powers and duties conferred or imposed on the Minister, under the Ministry of Health Act 1919, and the duties imposed by the Committee of the Privy Council for Medical Research, under the third act, the Minister may conduct or assist by grants or otherwise, any person to conduct research into any matters relating to the causation, prevention, diagnosis or treatment of illness or mental defectiveness.

It was only in 1963–1964 that the Ministry of Health began to support R&D in a wider context. Until then, it had regarded its research responsibilities as confined to the field of public health and the Zuckerman Report on 'Hospital Scientific and Technical Services', published in 1968, was concerned mainly with public health.[23]

Since the late 1950s the Department of Health in agreement with the Medical Research Council had also operated a small but growing decentralised scheme of grants for the support of minor projects of hospital organised research. This was partly undertaken through the locally organised clinical research scheme referred to above. Apart from that, there was only a small discretionary fund amounting to about £2500 per annum – a relic of what had been at the disposal of Sir John Simon in the late nineteenth century – that the Chief Medical Officer could use to initiate research.

At the beginning of the 1960s – that is, about 15 years after the establishment of the NHS – the capability and ability for research relevant to developments within the NHS were somewhat limited. There was no central research organisation and no general provision for research related to the running of the NHS. A number of enquiries in reports began to question the need for the development of such research but this had usually been done by outside experts who gave advice without necessarily having been given a clear research brief. The Ministry of Health began to look at its own activities at this time and to collect some research data. In addition it established a small research unit to look at developments within the NHS. This informal, semi-structured method of operation began to change in 1961. This was partly because of the need to produce statistical and other measures of efficiency as a result of publication in 1956 of the Guillebaud Report on the cost of the NHS[24] but also because of the organisation and beginnings of a hospital building programme and the need to develop knowledge about what capacity and equipment for operations would be required in the future.

In 1960 Sir George Godber (1908–2009) was appointed Chief Medical Officer. He had the vision to see that his Ministry needed to be able to answer a wider variety of questions related to the delivery of health care and improvements in health beyond the existing research on infectious disease and environmental hazards conducted by the Public Health Laboratory Service. Although good relations existed with the Medical Research Council, there were undoubtedly a number of conflicts between the Ministry and the Medical Research Council, and the latter was not really equipped to undertake the broad investigation of questions related to developments in health care.

Dr R.H.L. (Dick) Cohen (1907–1998) was the third Secretary of the Medical Research Council at that time and became concerned with the need to develop more applied research to improve NHS services. The Medical Research Council's priorities, however, lay in the advancement of medical knowledge rather than in the delivery of health care. Godber was able to persuade Cohen to transfer from the Medical Research Council to the Ministry of Health as Deputy Chief Medical Officer and to become responsible for developing research relevant to the NHS.

The administrator responsible for the operation of a sector of the Ministry called Organisation and Methods was John Cornish. Cornish had been in the Navy before joining the Ministry of Health as a Principal and during the Second World War had been involved in operational research on how to combat the threat to the UK from U-boats. He was thus very sympathetic to the development of research related to the functioning of a service.

The Department of Health's activities at this time were somewhat haphazard and not particularly well organised. Under Dr Cohen's direction, a Medical Research branch was established with Dr J.M.G. (Max) Wilson (1913–2006) and John Cornish responsible for encouragement and development of research. Wilson, a physician, had been trained in clinical medicine, including medical research, and had spent some years in charge of medical services to a number of tea plantations in India. Godber had recognised that although a certain number of enquiries, such as the analysis of statistical data, could only be done within the Ministry, research relating to matters concerned with health care, particularly the changing nature and the improvements in the organisation, planning and prioritisation of services, would be unlikely to have the support of those responsible for the delivery of services if it was only carried out internally. Godber, therefore, accepted the need to establish research commissioned by the Department of Health, but independent of it.

Organisational matters were under the direction of Mr Wolf Rudoe (b. 1916), Director of Statistics, and he became head of the research division with Wilson and Cornish accountable to him. Much of their activity was concerned with social security rather than with health services. Cohen stated that:[13]

> the paramount need for an executive department to establish from the outset, unassailable credentials of quality and independence in research is always uppermost in our minds and would by itself have been enough to lead us to try to place most of the work extramurally in departments of acknowledged reputation. Under these arrangements, a variety and quality and independence of thought would be brought to bear on NHS problems which could not be enlisted in any other way. Moreover, the possibility was open further ahead of secondments, or part time appointments, between research centres and the Department to their mutual benefit in education in each others problems and ways of thought.

Cohen also emphasised that there were, at least in medicine, researchers with a spontaneous interest in practical health service questions, as well as scientific journals able to assess and disseminate research results and a profession accustomed to combining an interest in research with a responsibility for providing a service. Difficulties in establishing HSR were certainly foreseen by its originators – Cohen, Godber, Wilson and others – but the prime focus of the specialty was conceived to be in social medicine and the UK was its cradle. There was a serious shortage of workers in the field and a real need to promote and develop this type of research that could not be satisfied by the current workforce or organisation. Part of the problem was the poor career prospects in social medicine and epidemiology, and the Department of Health recognised that, at least for a transitional period, it would have to provide additional respectable jobs in this field. There were also other constraints such as the differential salary scales between epidemiology, social medicine and clinical medicine. Clinical medicine had about a 20–30 per cent advantage in terms of salary at every level, since epidemiology and social medicine were considered as preclinical and not clinical subjects.

The Medical Research Council, to some extent, accepted that there was a need to develop a corpus of researchers in this area and in 1958 it awarded a number of senior clinical research fellowships – for example, to George Knox (b. 1926) in Birmingham and to myself (b. 1929) at St Thomas' Hospital in London.

Cohen recognised that the difficulty was going to be even greater in the development of social science, as well as in management and operational research, and a few pioneering individuals needed to be identified and stimulated to undertake such research at a time when there was no social science research council. In his view, the greatest need was for health economists, described by him as being 'the shyest birds'. One of the first economists attracted to the field of HSR in the UK was an American, Martin Feldstein (b. 1939), a researcher at Oxford who was persuaded to become involved in various health-related topics, such as the need for a community care hospital. It was not until the early 1970s, however, that a number of other individuals and a viable structure emerged. A conference was arranged by Professor Alan Williams (1912–1995) at York to discuss what part economists might play. Williams, a Professor of Economics at York, had been seconded previously to work in the Department of Education and from there had gone for a brief time to work in the Department of Health where he was influenced by R.H.L. (Dick) Cohen to become interested in the problems of HSR. As a result, Williams returned to York University to found a Department of Health Economics and Centre for Health Economics that has flourished there since that time. His major interest was in trying to develop a measure of the value of health – quality adjusted life years (QUALYs) – which could be used to value the importance of different health measures. The department at York became a unidisciplinary unit concerned with training and research in health economics and has produced such eminent health economists as Professor Tony Culyer (b. 1942) and Professor Alan Maynard (b. 1944).

The scale of activity of HSR at the beginning was relatively small.[19] The DHSS had £5.5 million for R&D. Of this, between one-quarter and one-third was spent on HSR, mainly on research units. The remainder was disbursed in the form of project grants, including locally organised clinical research. A much larger amount was available for capital development (£1.6 million), equipment, supply and appliance research (£1.5 million), and building and engineering work (£680 000). The research units, usually established in academic departments, hospitals or other research centres, were given broad terms of reference and a contract for seven years to deal with particular areas, such as drug addiction.

At the outset in 1970 there were eight units (Table 3.1). These were as follows: The Social Medicine and Health Services Research Unit at St Thomas' Hospital Medical School under myself (b. 1929); The Wolfson Institute of Chemical Technology under Professor Tom Whitehead (1923–2005); The Addiction Research Unit, jointly with the Medical Research Council, under Dr Griffiths Edwards (b. 1928); The Unit in Epidemiology and Medical Care, jointly with the Medical Research Council, under Dr Tom Meade (b. 1936); The Institute of Biometry and Community Medicine under Professor John Ashford (1929–2011) and Dr Norman Pearson (b. 1926); The Hospital Organisation Research Unit under Professor Martin Jacques (1917–2003); The Community Care Research Unit under Professor David Newell (b. 1929) and Dr John Walker (b. 1928); and The Special Hospitals Research Unit under Professor T.C.N.B. Gibbens and Dr T.G. Tennent.

Table 3.1   Health Service Research Units in 1970

Unit	Director
Social Medicine and Health Services Research Unit St Thomas' Hospital Medical School, London	Professor Walter Holland
Wolfson Institute of Chemical Technology Birmingham University and Hospital	Professor Tom Whitehead
Addiction Research Unit (joint with Medical Research Council) Institute of Psychiatry, Maudsley Hospital, London	Dr Griffiths Edwards
Unit in Epidemiology and Medical Care (joint with Medical Research Council) Northwick Park Hospital, Harrow	Dr Tom Meade

Unit	Director
Institute of Biometry and Community Medicine	Professor John Ashford
University of Exeter	Dr Norman Pearson
Hospital Organisation Research Unit Brunel University, London	Professor Martin Jacques
Community Care Research Unit University of Newcastle	Professor David Newell Dr John Walker
Special Hospitals Research Unit	Professor T.C.N.B. Gibbens
Institute of Psychiatry, London	Dr T.G. Tennent

The staff of these research centres or units were employees of the universities or parent organisations and subject to their terms and conditions of service. The DHSS provided a guaranteed level of support for a period of five to seven years under a formal contract with the host institution and the director. The scope and content of a unit's work was guided by an advisory committee on which the DHSS was represented and which included outside experts. Subject to the DHSS's right to comment on a report in draft, there was the normal freedom to publish at the Directors' discretion and this was fully maintained for many years. The terms and conditions of the environment and work for each of the units varied to some extent. The unit at St Thomas' Hospital, for example, had a specific remit to develop training in HSR that was not included in any of the unit contracts elsewhere. In addition to these units, there were a large number of programmes and project grants which are listed in *Portfolio for Health Volume 2*, published in 1973.[25]

By the early 1970s, in addition to the first eight units, two more were established – one at Kent and the second at Brunel University, concerned with social services organisation. Initial programmes of research undertaken by these units, as well as the programmes of research, are also fully listed in *Portfolio for Health Volume 2*.[25]

There was no clear organisation at the beginning. Units were given a great deal of freedom to formulate their own research programmes and to develop appropriate methods of operation. The budget of each unit was relatively limited when compared with present day levels. At St Thomas' Hospital, for example, we had an annual income of about £120 000. The directors of the original units were not paid from the research grant. They were honorary directors, paid by the universities or hospitals, and the research money was used to pay for additional research and support staff. An important point negotiated and accepted, without question, was the freedom to publish research findings. Draft publications had to be submitted to the DHSS who had four weeks to make comments. These could be taken into account but could also be ignored. As will be seen later, this condition was important for the integrity of the research but was on occasion also a source of conflict.

Cohen was concerned with the use of research findings. Steps were introduced to make certain that important results of departmental research would be publicly and critically assessed in the light of all other relevant information and then used as appropriate. The researchers were encouraged to publish in the scientific press and to present their findings at academic meetings. The DHSS thus derived authority from the work itself as well as the reputation of its authors, and the researchers were encouraged to find acknowledgement by competition with others. The DHSS's main role was to help: 'create the opportunity and machinery for discussion and consequent action, as for instance by subsidising publication where necessary and encouraging meetings concerned with HSR'.[13] Cohen recognised the danger that results considered valid, useful and important would not get fully disseminated or understood by those who should use and apply the research findings. Close links were to be established between those responsible for research and those responsible for the service within the DHSS and also in regional, area and district health authorities, in the hope that this would encourage the process of dissemination and interpretation. Perhaps one of the most important provisos, in the light of what has occurred since the start of this programme, was Cohen's statement that:

> there is only very little that can be said with assurance about the future. Whatever happens it is impossible for the Department to mark time in research. As we have already said, the Department in its planning and policy-making, cannot leave research into the value and management of potential new advances to the chance interest of others with no service responsibilities. If it does shift the onus in this way and the work is not done in time, it will have to act in default of the evidence. Nor can the Department abdicate its responsibility foreseeing that the public gets the aids and appliances it needs, for example, artificial limbs, hearing aids, or invalid vehicles. It seems likely however, that the next two or three years will be taken up with the health side, more with consolidation and development of existing research resources, than with expansion.[19]

Cohen considered that the first two years of the R&D programme would be spent in building up a research programme and consolidating and reinforcing the research being undertaken, rather than being concerned with changes in administration. Unfortunately this wish was not accomplished in the way that he would have liked. The most important reason for this – outside the remit of any of those involved in the foundation of the research programme – was the change in economic and political circumstances at the beginning of the 1970s, for example, the 'oil shock' and the restriction in research expenditure. There was also a lack of staff interest in the research and its direction within the DHSS and a failure of communication between researchers and officials.

The researchers themselves wanted to establish their own credibility within the academic environment and tended to be more concerned with undertaking research that was credible to their academic peers than research clearly relevant to the DHSS . Not all of the units had close relationships with the NHS. The closest relationship was probably at St Thomas' Hospital where every member of the research unit had an honorary appointment with the hospital and there was good coordination of activities between the two organisations.

The work originally started at St Thomas' Hospital was largely concerned with questions raised by the NHS administration on which it needed advice. The administration recognised the need to develop effective liaison between the researchers and the health and clinical administrators. Almost from the start, therefore, a health service manager, John Wyn Owen (b. 1942), was appointed jointly by the administration and the research unit to act as a link between the two. Finance for this was provided by the Research Endowment Fund of the hospital and the Kings' Fund who were interested in developing opportunities for administrators at that time.[26, 27] Unfortunately, with the changes in structure of the health service in 1974 and the restriction in the development of the NHS from around the middle of the 1970s until the end of the twentieth century, the initial appointment was not renewed.

At St Thomas' Hospital, however, close links between the NHS administration and the research unit continued and the link between clinical medicine and the research unit was also fostered through the joint honorary appointments. The Director of the Unit, for example, was a member of the Physicians Committee as were all his senior consultant level medical staff. This was not necessarily the case in other units where, to some extent at least, researchers pursued their own agendas. The problem of administration of research became an important issue in its own right and certainly led to some of the blocks in the development and application of HSR.

Perhaps the clearest example of the divide between those responsible for research at ministerial level in the Department of Health and those undertaking the research was in relation to studies on defining the needs and functions of the new district general hospitals. These were planned for Frimley and Bury St Edmunds on the principle that most health care would take place in the community. As mentioned earlier, at the original meeting to discuss the project, a very senior government official raised the issue of whether the DHSS could fund research that might question departmental policy. The researchers, supported by the Chief Scientist, insisted that it was the function of research to examine policy. It was agreed that this issue needed to be resolved at ministerial level and it took about six months before it was agreed that part of the function of research was indeed to question and evaluate policy that had already been determined. It became clear that Department officials were very uncomfortable with this concept and it has taken many years for the suspicion that existed between those responsible for policy and those concerned with research to subside and for the former to accept that researchers might query some of the policies that had been or were being developed.

Pioneers of Health Services Research

The development of the HSR programme by the Department of Health came about largely because of the recognition by Sir George Godber, the Chief Medical Officer, of the need for such research,[28, 29] and in this he was firmly backed by Gordon McLachlan (1918–2007), Secretary of the Nuffield Provincial Hospitals Trust. The Nuffield Trust (as it is now known) was founded as the Nuffield Provincial Hospitals Trust in 1940 by Viscount Nuffield (1877–1963) who recognised that there was a need to support health services outside London. The complementary organisation for London was the Kings' Fund established in honour of the coronation of Edward VII. Histories of the two voluntary charitable foundations have been documented.[30, 31] The Nuffield Provincial Hospitals Trust became interested in the development and planning of health services and it helped to fund a review of the services provided outside London. It also helped to establish the Emergency Bed Service and recognised the need for a regional organisation of emergency medical services during the Second World War, on which the NHS modelled its development in 1948.

McLachlan, who served as Secretary of the Trust from 1956 to 1986, was born in Leith in 1918 and his most important training was on the financial side of Scottish Local Government. He was articled to the City Chamberlain of the Edinburgh Corporation and grew up with the abiding stamp of that administrative methodology as stated by Edgar Williams, Chairman of the Trust. After war service as a gunnery officer in the

Royal Navy, during which McLachlan played rugby-football for the United Services, he entered the NHS early in its history. From 1948 to 1953, he was Deputy Treasurer of the North West Metropolitan Regional Hospital Board and then went as an accountant to the Nuffield Foundation. The Nuffield Provincial Hospitals Trust was founded initially under the umbrella of the Nuffield Foundation. Early on, however, it sought independence with the backing of two major figures in its early days – A.Q. Wells (1896–1956), first chairman of the Oxford Regional Board, and Sir Ernest Rock Carling (1877–1960). It was not long before the Trust, with Gordon McLachlan as its Secretary, moved from Nuffield Lodge to 3 Prince Albert Road, London. To his unique task, McLachlan brought financial probity, imaginative dynamism and a deeply emotional belief in the NHS. He had an uncanny knack of being able to identify problems that required enquiry and discussion and it is impossible to overestimate the contribution that he made to the promotion of HSR in the UK. Funds available to the Trust for supporting research on its own were miniscule. McLachlan called together groups of researchers, as well as those responsible for the delivery of health services and policy decisions at a central, regional and local level, and stimulated them to support research and become interested in it. He was outstanding in fomenting a climate of enquiry and questioning for the development of health services. Most of the work was done through publications, informal meetings, as well as providing seed money to a few individuals to start a particular area of research. McLachlan had a large number of contacts and relationships with influential people, such as Sir George Godber. He was apolitical and most of his influence was on civil servants and health professionals rather than politicians. His history of the Nuffield Trust shows how the Trust was able to capitalise on getting together people with common interest to undertake appropriate research.[30]

Godber himself was, of course, crucial to the development of HSR. He was one of the most outstanding Chief Medical Officers in the UK and attracted great respect in the medical profession as well as among his peer administrators and politicians. His ability to attract good people to work with him is legendary.

One of these was Dr R.H.L. (Dick) Cohen, another J.M.G. (Max) Wilson. Cohen was the individual who put in place the necessary organisation for the research programme within the Department of Health and was trusted by those in Government, in universities and in research councils so that the enterprise became successful. Max Wilson was a quiet and gentle individual who had great determination and intellect. He was able to identify the necessary problems for investigations and, in his personal relationships, to sustain, help and facilitate research. One of the best known aspects of this was his expertise and initiative in screening, where he wrote one of the fundamental monographs on the subject after a visit to the US.[32]

The organisation established by Cohen, Wilson and Cornish needed a Chief Scientist. The first Chief Scientist was Cohen himself who also became Deputy Chief Medical Officer and represented research at the highest levels within the DHSS. Through his administrative position as Deputy Chief Medical Officer, Cohen understood the research that was required, but was also able to influence those responsible for the development of policy to take note of research findings.

When Cohen retired as Chief Scientist in 1973, he was succeeded by Douglas Black (1913–2003), an eminent clinician who had been Professor of Medicine at Manchester. Black had done medical research and was particularly well known for his work on renal disease. Black's attitude towards research was perhaps best recounted in his Rock Carling lecture.[33] He was concerned not so much with the implementation of research as with the identification of possible research subjects and felt that his role was of an advisory nature. He chaired and participated in a variety of meetings identifying appropriate subjects for research and was involved and concerned with the quality and standards of the research commissioned.

As an academic, Black was not particularly comfortable within the Department of Health. This was partly because he was not entirely sympathetic to the bureaucratic nature of the Department and partly because, although his intellect and ability were well recognised, he was not trusted by the civil service administrators as Cohen had been, because he was not 'one of them'. Nevertheless, Black's time in the Department of Health was extremely important in terms of the establishment of a research ethos and of research capability. He did not have as high an opinion of his own accomplishments as many had from the outside and, when he was elected President of the Royal College of Physicians, he was glad to resign from his post as Chief Scientist in 1977.

Reviewing the many papers that exist regarding the origins of the OCS at the record office at Kew, it is interesting to see what concerned the administrators. Voluminous papers record the individuals able to attend meetings with Douglas Black. There are innumerable discussions on the accommodation and meals to be had by participants at the meetings. The records available on discussions of research, however, are rather fewer in number. The papers demonstrate the division between the medical side, as led by Black, and the administrative side as to what was important. The officials opposed several of Black's ideas and attempted to block some of the initiatives. Even though the research expertise in the Department, as well as outside, was largely medical at this time, the administrators favoured the addition of a strong body of social scientists to decision-making on research, perhaps to dilute the more scientific aspects of medicine!

Godber was succeeded in 1973 as Chief Medical Officer by Henry Yellowlees (1919–2006) who had been his Deputy. Yellowlees did not have Godber's enormous presence and credibility at all levels nor a sympathetic attitude towards HSR. His previous career had been in a regional hospital board and psychiatry and he had not been as involved in the development of research as Godber had been. Yellowlees' contacts outside the Department of Health were perhaps somewhat less thorough and influential than those of Godber who had been involved in the establishment of the NHS. His interest in research was not as great and Black was left to fight his own battles as Chief Scientist. As well as being a Professor of Medicine at Manchester, Black had also been a member of the Medical Research Council and had been particularly active in that body as Chairman of the Clinical Research Board. There was thus a close relationship between the Medical Research Council and the Department of Health R&D activities.

In 1978 Black was followed as Chief Scientist by Professor Arthur Buller (b. 1923). Buller's background was completely different. He had been a Professor of Physiology, first at St Thomas' Hospital Medical School and then at Bristol University where he had been elected Dean of the Medical School. Buller had served on the Medical Research Council and had a good knowledge of medical research. But his major strength was on research of the nervous system where he had made important discoveries on nerve pathways and neurological activity and he was not a clinician. When at St Thomas' Buller had done some work with Professor Sharpey-Schafer (1908–1963), as a Senior Lecturer, but this was not a major clinical commitment. Buller's major concern was not in the identification of new research areas, but in the improvement, in his view, of the quality of HSR. He perceived that much of the research had been undertaken by the large number and variety of researchers from the social sciences, as well as social medicine and clinical medicine, and considered that this was not of as high a calibre as that undertaken by physiologists or basic scientists. Buller was determined to improve both the quality and standing of the research funded by the Department of Health. He epitomised many of the prejudices against HSR which he considered to be a 'soft' subject. When appointed, he was not the only candidate put forward for the job. The other candidate is said to have been Professor A.C. Dornhorst (1915–2003), Professor of Medicine at St

George's Hospital Medical School and, like Buller, on the Medical Research Council Clinical Research Board. It is rumoured that Buller was chosen largely because he was considered to have had administrative experience as Dean of a Medical School although he had only held the post for about a year and thus his knowledge of administration was not necessarily as great as that of the people who selected him!

Buller was Chief Scientist at a time of great change in politics. The Conservative Government had taken over after Callaghan's Government had been defeated in the General Election. There was a change in the political climate towards HSR and research in general and Buller reflected some of these pressures. He tried to impose a somewhat different structure on HSR than his predecessor. His major concern was the quality of research and he introduced a far more stringent method of appraisal, both of research units as well as individual research programmes. This resulted in a number of tensions, not helped by Buller's inflexible personality.

One of Buller's major aims had been to return the Rothschild money to the Medical Research Council. He felt more akin to basic than applied research and was somewhat sceptical of the ethos of applied research in epidemiology, HSR and the social sciences. He attempted to strengthen his role within the Department of Health through the appointment of a Deputy Chief Scientist, expert in HSR, and approached me to fulfil this role, at least part-time. Unfortunately, however, I was already committed to spend six months at the University of California, Los Angeles, on sabbatical and was unwilling to take on administrative responsibilities within the Department of Health. A basic scientist was, therefore, appointed as deputy to undertake the administrative duties while Buller was able to concentrate on the scientific aspects.

In 1982 Buller was succeeded by Sir Desmond Pond (1919–1986) who had been a Professor of Psychiatry and was far more liberal minded and concerned with allaying the tensions that had begun to develop in HSR.

CONCLUSION

HSR was fortunate in the figures in positions of authority in the broader health field when it began. Godber, McLachlan, Cohen, Wilson and Cornish were, in their different ways, among those who understood its importance and championed its development. Black, first and foremost a clinician and academic, was not so well equipped to operate within the political and bureaucratic constraints of the civil service although he was crucial in establishing a research ethos and capability. Building on the work of predecessors like Haldane, Addison, Rothschild and Dainton, these giants strove to introduce concepts such as the measurement of need and the requirement of scientific evaluation into the planning and delivery of health services.

REFERENCES

1 Haldane Report (1918). Report of the Machinery of Government Committee, Ministry of Reconstruction. Cmnd 9230.
2 Haldane Report (1918), para. 56, p. 16.
3 Haldane Report (1918), para. 14, p. 6.
4 Haldane Report (1918), para. 57, p. 32.
5 Haldane Report (1918), para. 45, p. 29.
6 Haldane Report (1918), para. 42, p. 29.
7 Haldane Report (1918), para. 38, p. 28.
8 Haldane Report (1918), para. 74, p. 35.
9 National Health Service Act (1946).
10 Rothschild Report (1971). The organisation and management of Government R&D. In: *Cabinet Office: A Framework for Government Research and Development*. London: HMSO.
11 Ministry of Reconstruction (1919). Memorandum on the Future Organisation of Medical Research. London: HMSO.
12 Austoker, J. (1989). Walter Morley Fletcher and the origins of a basic biomedical research policy. In: Bryden, L. and Austoker, J. (eds), *Historical Perspectives on the Role of the Medical Research Council of the United Kingdom and its Predecessor, the Medical Research Committee, 1913–1953*. Oxford: Oxford University Press.
13 Cohen, R.H.L. (1971). The role and programme of the DHSS in health services research. In: McLachlan, G. (ed.), *Portfolio for Health 1: Problems and Progress in Medical Care. 6th Series. Essays on Current Research*. London: Oxford University Press for the Nuffield Provincial Hospitals Trust.
14 Committee of Enquiry into the Organisation of Civil Science (1963). *Report of the Committee of Enquiry into the Organisation of Civil Science, under the Chairmanship of Sir Burke Trend*. Cmnd 2171. London: HMSO.
15 McLachlan, G. (ed.) (1978). *Five Years After: A Review of Health Care Research Management after Rothschild*. Oxford: Oxford University Press.
16 Dainton Report (1971). The future of the Research Council System. In: *Cabinet Office: A Framework for Government Research and Development*. London: HMSO.
17 *Cabinet Office* (1972). *Framework for Government Research and Development*. Presented to Parliament by the Lord Privy Seal by Command of Her Majesty, July. London: HMSO.
18 Kogan, M., Henkel, M. and Hanney, S. (2006). *Government and Research: Thirty Years of Evolution*. Second edition. Dordrecht: Springer.

19   Cohen, R.H.L. (1971). The department's role in research and development.
     In: McLachlan, G. (ed.), *Portfolio for Health 1. Problems and Progress in
     Medical Care. 6th Series. Essays on Current Research.* London: Oxford
     University Press for the Nuffield Provincial Hospitals Trust.
20   Black, D. (1974). Organization of health services research. *British Medical
     Bulletin*, **30**(3), 199–202.
21   Taylor, D. and Teeling-Smith, G. (1984). *Health Services, UK Science
     Policy. A Critical Review of Policies for Publicly Funded Research.* London
     and New York: Longman.
22   Holland, W.W. (2009). Personal communication (a participant at the meet-
     ing).
23   Zuckerman Report (1968). Hospital Scientific and Technical Services.
     London: HMSO.
24   Guillebaud Report (1956). Cost of the National Health Service: Report of
     the Committee of Enquiry. London: HMSO.
25   McLachlan, G. (ed.) (1973). *Portfolio for Health 2: The Developing
     Programme of the DHSS in Health Services Research. Problems and
     Progress in Medical Care. 8th Series. Essays on Current Research.* London:
     Oxford University Press for the Nuffield Provincial Hospitals Trust.
26   Owen, J.W. (1978). The difficulties of linking administration to community
     medicine and to health services – St Thomas' experience. *World Hospitals*,
     14(1), 38.
27   Owen, J.W. and Holland, W.W. (1976). Research and administration: the
     uneasy relationship. In: Dunnell, K. (ed.), *Health Services Planning.* King
     Edward's Hospital Fund for London, pp. 28–32.
28   Sheard, S. and Donaldson, L. (2006). *The Nation's Doctor. The Role of the
     Chief Medical Officer 1855–1998.* Nuffield Trust. Oxford: Radcliffe Pub-
     lishing.
29   Webster, C. (1996). *The Health Services Since the War. Volume II. Govern-
     ment and Health Care: The British National Health Service 1958–1979.*
     London: HMSO.
30   McLachlan, G. (1992). *A History of the Nuffield Provincial Hospitals Trust,
     1940–1990.* London: Nuffield Provincial Hospitals Trust.
31   Maxwell, R. and Granshaw, L. (1987). *The King's Fund: Yesterday, Today
     and Tomorrow.* London: King Edward VII's Hospital Fund for London.
32   Wilson, J.M.G. and Jungner, G. (1968). *Principles and Practice of Screen-
     ing for Disease.* Geneva: World Health Organisation.
33   Black, D. (1984). *An Anthology of False Antitheses.* London: Nuffield
     Provincial Hospitals Trust.

4. Personal reflections

BEGINNINGS

I entered St Thomas' Hospital Medical School from school in 1947 with four A-Levels in Botany, Zoology, Chemistry and Physics, rather more than the equivalent of a first MB. The Secretary of the Medical School, Dr A.L. Crockford (1897–1992) considered that it was unnecessary for me to repeat the course for the first MB and arranged for me to work with Dr Tom Day, a Reader in Pathology, as his laboratory assistant. Day, a charismatic individual, was an outstanding pathologist and was doing research on connective tissue. I was involved in preparing the rat preparations for the examination of collagen and the 'ground matter' binding it to the skin.[1,2] One year with Tom Day introduced me to the attractions and challenges of medical research.

At the end of the first year, when I entered the second MB course with my contemporaries, my aim was to become involved in medical research. I did reasonably well in the examination and was selected to do a BSc. I chose to do this in Physiology, with Professor Henry Barcroft (1904–1998), Dr Maureen Young and Dr Charles Vass among others. There were four of us on this course that introduced us to many research methods. We were involved in various research initiatives, including the measurement of oxygen and blood CO_2 for the cardiologists and cardiac surgeons.[3] This exposure to research philosophy and methods contributed to my involvement in and enthusiasm for medical research, especially on physiological systems.

I became fascinated by aspects of child health and paediatrics, and on qualification, I started work with Dr Maureen Young, Reader in Physiology, whose special interest was neonatal medicine. I began a study to ascertain the levels of blood pressure in newborn babies, to see whether, by the measurement of blood pressure, it was possible to identify those babies at particular risk of death. I was also interested in the reactivity of the vascular systems of newborns. My first three clinical appointments were in casualty, medicine (on the medical unit) and the children's department at St Thomas' Hospital (1955–1956) and I was able to be present at deliveries in the obstetric wards of the hospital. I arranged with the midwives to be called to attend all deliveries on certain nights to measure the blood pressure of the newborn babies and the reactivity of their vascular systems. With Dr Young I published a number of papers on this subject.[4-6] Undertaking this paediatric research gave me training in research methods, as well as clinical medicine.

Since I had entered Medical School direct from school, I had not done National Service but was expected to do this after attaining full registration – that is, after two house officer appointments. Because of my experience in physiological research, the Professor of Physiology, Henry Barcroft, had negotiated with the Royal Air Force (RAF) that I should be posted to the Institute of Aviation Medicine in Farnborough to participate in some of the physiological work taking place there. I was called up after my third house officer post and entered the RAF in August 1956, at the time of the Suez Crisis. This meant that all personnel were needed for operational stations rather than research. I was posted as a Medical Officer at a RAF station in Coltishall in Norfolk and was there for three months. I had relatively little to do, since I was looking after 2000–3000 very fit young individuals.

In December 1956, I received a telephone call from the Medical Director of the personnel branch of the Air Ministry inviting me to consider another job in the Central Public Health Laboratory of the Public Health Laboratory Service (PHLS) involving the measurement of respiratory function.

The RAF was concerned with respiratory infections, particularly in recruits. Adenovirus infection is extremely common in young adults and this was causing high morbidity in the recruit training camps. A vaccine against adenovirus infection had been developed recently in the US and it was intended to carry out a randomised controlled trial of this vaccine to be produced by Glaxo in the UK, under the aegis of the PHLS, with a RAF Medical Officer in charge. The individual who had been recruited to do this had developed tuberculosis and they were faced with a vacancy that had to be filled at short notice. I was selected for the task because my personnel records showed that I had more clinical experience than any of my contemporaries, in view of my deferment, I had experience of research with an additional research degree, and most importantly, I owned a car! This was clearly going to be much more interesting than being an underemployed Station Medical Officer.

Christmas intervened between my acceptance of the post and the start of the trial scheduled for mid to end January 1957. Unfortunately, however, the scientists at Glaxo left the incubator on over the Christmas holiday and the trial vaccine samples were rendered useless. In January 1957, therefore, I was at the Central Public Health Laboratory working with Dr Corbett McDonald (b. 1918), ready to carry out a large scale randomised controlled trial of a new vaccine but this had failed its safety test. I was not in limbo for long. That month, Professor Tommy Francis (1900–1969) – an epidemiologist from Ann Arbor, Michigan – on a visit to Hong Kong, identified a new influenza virus that was likely to reach the US and Europe later that year. The PHLS was informed. Dr McDonald was involved in respiratory virus investigations and was very interested. He suggested that the RAF was a suitable milieu to undertake surveillance to determine when the influenza virus would reach the UK. The Director of Hygiene and Research, Air Vice-Marshal Wilson, decided that the RAF would be willing to act with the Medical Research Council and the PHLS as a test bed for developing surveillance for the new influenza virus.

I was given the choice of going back to being Medical Officer of a station which I had found rather dull, doing what had originally been intended – namely, going to work on physiology at the Institute of Aviation Medicine – or becoming involved with this new project. While continuing to work on physiology was attractive, it could be done at any time in the future whereas the investigation of a new influenza pandemic was novel and challenging and not likely to arise frequently. I opted to remain with the PHLS at Colindale.

In the 1950s, medical education did not include epidemiology. Over the next 18 months I learned about field epidemiology and developed a surveillance system for influenza in the RAF. I was thrown in at the deep end but was fortunate in that Dr Corbett McDonald was an enthusiastic and outstanding teacher. My time at the epidemiological research laboratory was fascinating. As well as establishing the surveillance system, I managed a randomised controlled trial to determine the effectiveness of a new influenza vaccine and undertook a study on the manifestations of influenza to try to see whether it was possible to distinguish influenza infection from other forms of acute respiratory infection in young adults.[7–11]

After my experience in the RAF, I returned in 1958 as a Lecturer in Medicine and Registrar to the Medical Unit at St Thomas'. The Professor of Medicine at the time was E.P. Sharpey-Schafer (1908–1963), an extremely far-seeing individual who had been responsible for bringing St Thomas' into the twentieth century, stimulating medical research and enthusing many individuals to take up clinical research. I became one of the 'Schafer's boys', a talented group who attained many senior positions – for example, Professors S.J.G. Semple (b. 1926), A.C. Dornhorst (1915–2003), P.F.D. Naylor (1924–2009), A. Buller (b. 1923) and H.E. de Wardener (b. 1915). Schafer knew my interests and said that I could spend my year with him in any way I wanted. I had to carry out certain clinical tasks, such as outpatient and inpatient duties as a registrar, but I was also encouraged to begin to do research. His policy as Professor of Medicine was to offer a year in his department with opportunities for research. If an individual showed promise and enthusiasm, support continued. At this stage, I was not sure whether I wanted to do epidemiological research or was more interested in paediatrics. I, therefore, undertook three separate tasks – first, an epidemiological study of respiratory infection in hospital patients,[12] second, clinical research on respiratory infections in children and babies,[13] and finally, clinical medicine in adults as well as in children.[14]

It soon became clear that my main interest was in epidemiology which offered remarkable opportunities at that time. To pursue this specialty, however, I needed further qualifications and training in the field. The Medical Research Council was advertising Rockefeller research fellowships in the US. I applied for one and was interviewed by Sir Harold Himsworth (1905–1993), Secretary of the Medical Research Council, who made it clear he would support my application if it was concerned with paediatric and clinical research. But he would not support an application for training in epidemiology in the US because I needed basic training in epidemiology in this country first. On his advice, therefore, I applied for a Medical Research Council Senior Clinical Research Fellowship for training in the UK.

Applying for these fellowships was a complicated process. The medical school or institution sponsoring the applicant had to guarantee that at the end of the three-year training period, a consultant position would be available. St Thomas', therefore, had to guarantee that I would obtain a consultant post at senior lecturer level at the end of three years. My sponsors welcomed this possibility since there was as yet no epidemiological academic unit in the Medical School or Hospital. At all times during my period at St Thomas' I was encouraged and supported by the senior staff. St Thomas' had a reputation of being a stuffy, conservative institution but this was far from the case. It was, in fact, very forward looking and very supportive of its graduates if they wished to pursue an interest that might be of value to the institution in the future.

For training in the UK, the Medical Research Council decided that I would work at the London School of Hygiene and Tropical Medicine (LSHTM) with Professor Sir Austin Bradford Hill (1897–1991), a medical statistician and epidemiologist, Professor Sir Richard Doll (1912–2005) and Professor Donald Reid (1914–1977). I spent two years at the LSHTM and took part in a wide variety of investigations of the epidemiology of Down's Syndrome,[15] of chronic cardiorespiratory diseases[16, 17] and blood pressure.[18–20] I had no formal training in epidemiology, medical statistics or public health. I sat in on many courses and lectures but took no academic qualification in the subject. At first I worked with Doll on his investigation of chromosomal abnormalities and attended many consultations that Bradford Hill held with investigators to help them with medical statistics. I then transferred to work with Reid on his studies of chronic cardiorespiratory disease in post office and telephone workers. Reid decided that I should spend a year (1961–1962) in the US and negotiated with the Medical Research Council for a position at the Department of Epidemiology, at Johns Hopkins School of Hygiene. There I continued the work that I had been doing in London on chronic cardiorespiratory disease in telephone workers in the US and was thus able to carry out a comparative study in American and British workers to try to identify some of the causes of chronic respiratory disease.[21–4]

My year in the US allowed me to visit other key institutions in all parts of the country, including New York, Chicago, Los Angeles, San Francisco, Cincinnati, Denver and Birmingham (Alabama), both to find out about work in progress and to see how epidemiology was taught and practised in the US.[i] My travel was financed partly by funds from Johns Hopkins and partly by an allowance from St Thomas'. I was also fortunate to be appointed consultant to the US Division of Air Pollution Research of the National Institutes of Health which enabled me to visit a number of sites undertaking work on the influence of air pollution on respiratory disease.

St Thomas' appointed me Senior Lecturer in Social Medicine while I was still at Johns Hopkins, probably at least in part to encourage me to return to London. For many British visitors to the US in the early 1960s, the offer of posts and their attraction in terms of salary and facilities were very tempting. I wanted, however, to fulfil my obligations to St Thomas' and I also much preferred working in the UK, although the offer of several senior posts in epidemiology in the US did my morale no harm!

On my return to St Thomas' in October 1962, I took up my post as Senior Lecturer in Social Medicine in the Department of Medicine with the intention of developing epidemiology. St Thomas' Hospital had in 1961 appointed a new Chief Executive, Bryan McSwiney (1921–2011), known as the Clerk of Governors. One of the first problems he faced was the need to modernise the content and handling of medical records. The

---

[i] For a list of the institutions visited, please see the appendix at the end of this chapter.

use of computers was increasing and McSwiney wondered if they could be used in this context. He sought advice from one of the Ministry of Health's Medical Officers, Dr M.A. Heasman (1926–2000), who was responsible for information systems. Heasman advised McSwiney to wait for my return from Baltimore and then to seek my help. He knew I had performed research on medical records and, while in the US, had had considerable exposure to computers and the analysis of medical records, particularly at the University of California, Los Angeles which I had visited on a number of occasions.

Therefore, in late October 1962 Bryan McSwiney approached me. With the available computing facilities and knowledge, it did not seem feasible to computerise medical records in their entirety but it seemed practicable to computerise patient summaries and test results. The first step was to determine the availability and help of other medical colleagues, Edward De Bono (b. 1933), later of lateral thinking fame, and John Colley (b. 1930). Together we examined patient records and showed that to obtain a reasonable record of the course of illness, it would be necessary to create a pro-forma, improve doctors' handwriting and have access to the nurses' notes. It was also desirable to involve nurses, technicians, pharmacists, porters and medical record librarians to gain a complete account of patient experiences.

We also demonstrated the difficulties of using optical scanning to translate the records into a form suitable for computer analysis which proved far more difficult than expected. As well as the account published of this work,[25, 26] we wrote a confidential memorandum to the Ministry of Health to warn them about our unfortunate experiences with the computing firm used for this project. Imagine my surprise to find out subsequently that this firm had become the preferred contractor on several DHSS contracts. Some years later, on a train journey, I met the Under-Secretary who had handled these contracts. I enquired why this preferential status had been given after the report we had submitted. He replied: 'your letter was destroyed, on receipt, as it might have influenced future commercial policy' – an important lesson for a researcher about how decisions are made at the centre of government!

As a result of my initial working experience, I realised that epidemiological methods and principles could be applied to the health service. My appointment as a Senior Lecturer within the Department of Medicine, with responsibility for social medicine and epidemiology, enabled me to carry out epidemiological research as well as clinical work. Then, unfortunately, Professor Sharpey-Schafer died prematurely of cancer of the oesophagus. Before appointing a new Professor of Medicine, the Medical School decided that they would create a new department independent of medicine to secure the future of epidemiology and social medicine. This Department was responsible for teaching, service and research, and consisted of a medical statistician, a medically qualified epidemiologist, a social scientist and several field workers, all of whom had nursing or health visitor qualifications. This was done deliberately because one of the candidates for the Professorship was very antagonistic towards these particular specialties, and the Medical School did not wish to prejudice the development of the department to which they had committed themselves. I was thus made independent far more rapidly than had originally been envisaged and was faced with the development of an academic department without the protection of a senior professor. Fortunately, the Professor of Medicine eventually appointed – W.I. Cranston (1928–2007) – was sympathetic towards epidemiology so I did not have any serious difficulties.

My first studies with St Thomas' Unit built on my research in respiratory medicine. During my work in the RAF, I had become aware that respiratory infection and illness in young people could lead to permanent lung damage. The first group of studies was concerned with the development of respiratory disease and respiratory function in a cohort of newborn babies. I enlisted the help of the Medical Officer of Health for Harrow who agreed to a series of studies in his borough. We investigated the effect of factors such as social class and levels of air pollution on the development of respiratory infections and respiratory function in newborn babies, by identifying and visiting all births in six electoral wards of Harrow between 1963–1965; the wards were specifically chosen to reflect different social and environmental conditions. The babies were visited within six weeks of birth by a fieldworker, a questionnaire was completed and the baby examined. A one in six sample of babies was visited again either by myself or by Professor John Colley. We established the ventilatory function of the baby within six weeks of birth by measuring, on a specially developed instrument, inspiratory and expiratory volume and inspiratory and expiratory flow rates on crying. In total about 2500 families were visited over a two-year period by our team and were followed until the child reached the age of five years. At each annual visit, the ventilatory function of those infants who had been measured within the first six weeks of life was measured again. The other five-sixths of the sample had annual visits where details of respiratory illnesses and growth were recorded. We were able to obtain an idea of the development of respiratory disease from birth. We had details of prenatal events as well, and were able to show that the most important factors in the development of respiratory illnesses in five-year-olds were the occurrence of respiratory illnesses in the first year of life and smoking by parents. This was also true for ventilatory function which was also lower in those infants who had an illness in the first year of life and was also affected by the number of illnesses in the first five years of life.[27–33]

The second series of studies (1964–1973) was concerned with children from the age of five years and over. For this I obtained the help of the County Medical Officer for Kent and chose four different areas of the county (Rochester; Malling rural district; Cranbrook, Tenterden and Romney Marsh rural districts; and Tonbridge), illustrating different social and environmental factors. We used the routine examinations of children at ages five, nine, 11 and 13 years to collect data on respiratory illnesses and ventilatory function.[34–6] At that time, the Medical Officers of Health in places like Kent and Harrow were influential and had access to resources such as qualified nurses. They were keen to cooperate in academic research and were only too willing to help in the development of studies on the epidemiology of respiratory disease in children. Funds for this research did not need to be very large because most of the manpower was already in place and most of the information could be obtained during routine examinations of the babies or schoolchildren. We were also able to get small sums of money to support the work from funds available from the Regional Board through locally organised clinical research. The Medical School had also provided me with the basis of a so-called 'well found' department by providing a statistician and fieldworkers.

These studies, which continued over a period of about ten years, were extremely fruitful. We were, for example, among the first workers to demonstrate the effect of passive smoking – that is, smoking by parents – on the frequency of respiratory illness and lung function in children, as well as the effect of smoking on the schoolchildren themselves.

With the reorganisation of the NHS in 1974 and the disappearance of Local Authority Departments of Public Health, such studies became increasingly difficult. The Directors of Public Health (formerly Medical Officers of Health) and their Community Physicians did not have access to the resources of their predecessors and these investigations became very much more expensive and difficult to undertake.

It is often forgotten that in the past, epidemiological research was in many ways very much easier than it is now because we were able to mobilise the assistance of people to undertake investigations, after appropriate training, within their routine work. All our studies depended on cooperation with local medical, nursing and other staff. Because I had been a medical student, house officer and registrar at St Thomas', I had performed clinical research and was considered to be a reasonably respectable clinician and St Thomas' Hospital and Medical School had committed themselves to provide a career for me and to foster what was then known as social medicine, after I had completed my training as a Medical Research Council Senior Clinical Research Fellow.

The commitment of St Thomas', considered by some to be the epitome of conservative London medicine, to what was then seen as a fringe subject was not surprising. The Institution had always been at the forefront of population medicine concerns and prided itself on looking after the health of the population of Lambeth. It was one of the first London medical schools to have an academic professorial department in medicine. Its alumni included Florence Nightingale as well as John Simon, the first equivalent of the Chief Medical Officer. There were also some consultants with traditional medical views, who, although they had private practices in Harley Street, held radical, progressive social views.

In developing the Department of Social Medicine and Clinical Epidemiology, it was essential to consider its future. Many individuals at that time – including Charles Fletcher (1911–1995), Donald Reid (1914–1977) and Geoffrey Rose (1926–1993) – were beginning to develop major disease-orientated research, for example, in respiratory and cardiovascular disease. Relatively very few people, however, were concerned with studying health services. Clearly, St Thomas' required some research on health services to use both in rebuilding the hospital and in its management. The Clerk of the Governors acknowledged the importance of this and a series of population studies was planned to take place in Lambeth (see Chapter 6). Our aim was to identify the types of both community and hospital care necessary for the population to use in planning appropriate services. The Department of Health also encouraged the development of the IISR unit and I was able to continue both with epidemiological research on respiratory and cardiovascular disease, my own major interest, and to design and oversee a series of the HSR studies described later in the book.

ESTABLISHMENT OF HEALTH SERVICES RESEARCH AND OF CHIEF SCIENTISTS

As has already been described, the Ministry of Health began to recognise the need for an independent research capacity in the 1960s. Until that time, most medical/health research was supported by the Medical Research Council whose major interest since its inception before the First World War was in basic research in practical subjects such as physiology, biochemistry, pharmacology and bacteriology.[37] During the First World War (1914–1918) it had become involved in a variety of relevant research problems – for example, the causes and prevention of 'trench foot'. After the end of the war, however, the Medical Research Council quickly became more interested again in basic questions rather than in the application of scientific findings. This can be best exemplified by the relatively few examples of notable advances in health research, as described in *Foundations for Health Improvement*.[38] The Medical Research Council's relatively poor performance in applied research is illustrated by the absence of any separate Board concerned with clinical research within the organisation until 1953.[37]

The Nuffield Provincial Hospitals Trust (now the Nuffield Trust) Secretary was Gordon McLachlan. He was a visionary who recognised the need for applied research to look at the services to be provided by the developing NHS.[39] The Trust did not have a large endowment but the small amount of this free research money was used very wisely in two main ways. The first was to develop small research projects that could then be taken forward by the national authorities with much larger financial research resources and to hold informal seminars and discussions that would bring together both researchers, providers and administrators to identify crucial areas of exploration. The second was to develop an 'intelligence' system/function that would help in the identification, development and support of research topics. Godber, Cohen and McLachlan were a formidable trio who were able to work together to sustain and develop a real research capacity for the NHS. Unfortunately such a visionary group has never been replicated.

On retirement in 1973, Cohen was succeeded by Douglas Black, a very distinguished physician who had been Professor of Medicine in Manchester.[40] He was a close colleague and successor of Robert Platt (1900–1978), who was the Professor of Medicine at Manchester and President of the Royal College of Physicians, and both were outstanding clinical researchers in renal medicine. Black had helped to establish the Clinical Research Board of the Medical Research Council. Godber also retired almost simultaneously, to be succeeded as Chief Medical Officer by Sir Henry Yellowlees who had risen from the ranks of administrative medicine of regional hospital administration. Yellowlees did not have Godber's background or interest in public health and was not as concerned to encourage HSR as his predecessor. Black was primarily a researcher and clinician, not an administrator. As Chief Scientist he saw himself as an adviser rather than being in operational control of the research function. Cohen, fortunately, in his role as Deputy Chief Medical Officer *and* Chief Scientist had established the research function on a firm footing in the largely administrative government department – which was not inbred with a research ethos and which has always found the research function irksome. Black did not enjoy his time in the DHSS, finding that his enquiring mind and mode of operation were severely trammelled by the administration of the government department which, imbued with the philosophy of the Civil Service, considered that its function was to administrate the NHS efficiently and to follow the wishes of its political masters.

It was at this time, the beginning of the 1970s, that the basic structure and direction of all government-funded research was reviewed and altered. The Conservative Government under Edward Heath took the view that much UK research was not concerned with the application of results and commissioned the Rothschild Report.[41] This, in essence, considered that about 25 per cent of all Research Council supported research required a *customer*. This principle was also to be adopted by research funded directly by all Departments of State. All funded research, therefore, had to tackle a practical question with an identifiable customer who would pay for the research and be responsible for applying the findings.

This principle was, as might have been expected, widely opposed by the scientific community. The principle of *customer–contractor* was readily applicable in sciences such as chemistry or engineering. In medicine, however, the problem was more complex. Many health service researchers and clinicians welcomed the principle of more and, hopefully, better applied research relevant to their interests and concerns, rather than those of the basic scientists who dominated the levers of research funding power. But in medicine trying to disentangle basic from applied research is difficult. In order to treat high blood pressure, for example, it is necessary to know about the mechanisms of blood pressure control (basic research) to develop relevant pharmacological or other agents that can be used in its treatment or prevention. It is also necessary to consider appropriate methods of service delivery, such as hospital or community services or population screening as opposed to opportunistic screening, as well as the various environmental, social or nutritional factors that can affect levels of pressure. Thus the dissociation of pure and applied research was and is a false distinction. There was no doubt that at that time the balance between basic and applied research needed to be altered – with a much greater emphasis on the latter – and the fact that researchers in *all* areas were of equal importance and value needed to be recognised.

Douglas Black was undoubtedly of major help in this transition of policy. As a clinician he recognised the importance of the application of HSR findings, but he also understood the need for basic research to underpin the clinical practice.

With the 'transfer' of a proportion of the Medical Research Council's budget to the service Department of Health, the latter needed to perform the customer function. The difficulty in this was two-fold. Most DHSS staff were career civil servants and the majority were arts graduates. The few medically qualified staff in the Department had no scientific or research background either and the same was true of other professional staff, such as nurses or therapists. Thus a great deal of disagreement, concern and disillusionment existed.

The Department tried to manage the change by the creation in 1972–1973 of the Office of the Chief Scientist (OCS) and the advent of Research Liaison Groups (RLGs). These were established in a number of specific areas that represented departmental policy groups – for example, children's services and forensic psychiatry. They were led by the relevant policy administrator, usually an assistant secretary, and staffed by administrators but usually including three appropriate scientific advisers. Their role was to identify research priorities, call for research bids to investigate one or more of these, and evaluate the bids. Kogan Korman and Henkel give a good description of the process and the problems.[42] The problems included the fact that the administrators were not willing participants, found great difficulties in developing a research agenda and did not consider the whole process to be a relevant use of their time and resources. The groups met rarely, changed personnel frequently, and, without any identifiable budget, had great difficulty in developing suitable research. The main difficulty was, however, that the specific topics for the groups did not include acute services (or subsets of these), planning or resource allocation – major topics of real concern to the Department of Health and its political masters – but concentrated on worthy, but minority interests, such as mental handicap or forensic psychiatry. Black and the research management team did their best to try to manage the process. But, in common with the rest of public services, they were faced with staff cuts, and were unable to make a success of the structure that had been imposed on them in response to the Rothschild Report by the external management consultants McKinsey. The independent evaluation by Kogan et al. was not encouraging![42]

At the same time Black and the OCS were continuing to commission and fund a variety of more general HSR. They strengthened a number of research units that had been created by Cohen and commissioned several new units, particularly in the social sciences.

Training

There was, however, one very major gap – the training of new researchers.

Although a number of units had been created, research funded and commissioned, there was no policy for training new researchers in HSR. Only the Unit at St Thomas's included the training of researchers and funding for trainees in its terms of reference. There were several difficulties. The Department of Health expected the universities to be responsible for education and training, and, in its funding policy, was unable to commit itself to the establishment of any career structure. It was bound by the Parliamentary funding system allocating funding for a limited defined period, usually three to five years. This was a cause of great concern – the equivalent organisation, the Medical Research Council, had the ability to promote staff, and to provide a career in research. They also had recognised junior and senior training fellowships.

Although Black and his colleagues recognised the need for training and a career structure they were unable to persuade the rest of the Department of Health or indeed the Government to create this. It was not generally recognised that HSR workers required specific training and a separate career structure. Those in this field came from a number of disciplines – medicine, sociology, economics and statistics. Of the medically qualified researchers, most had training and experience in epidemiology or public health. In most cases this type of research has to be multidisciplinary and this requires training and experience. Health economics alone retained its unidisciplinary function. Individuals who work in multidisciplinary units can risk losing their connection to the parent discipline. If they have not contributed to knowledge in their own specialty, they may also be at a disadvantage when applying for a professorial appointment.

The Unit at St Thomas' developed an elaborate system to ensure a continuing relationship with an individual's parent discipline and to make certain that the work included in any project was of an appropriate academic quality. To meet these needs within the academic environment of a Medical School, the Senior Social Scientist was encouraged to spend time with Professor Margot Jefferys (1916–1999) of the Department of Medical Sociology at Bedford College, the Senior Economist spent about two days per week in the Department of Social Administration with Professor Abel Smith (1926–1996) at The London School of Economics, and the Senior Statistician was attached to Professor Peter Armitage (b. 1924) at the LSHTM. These arrangements ensured that each discipline retained its links with their own specialty and helped to maintain the quality of HSR. The success of these arrangements can be measured by the subsequent careers of those coming to St Thomas' in their early professional lives. Many succeeded in attaining the highest ranks of their discipline in other universities or organisations such as the World Health Organisation and the Office of National Statistics. Unfortunately this model was not widely replicated and training and career structure have bedevilled HSR over many years.

Successors to Black

Cohen and Black had laid a sound foundation for HSR at the Department of Health and outside. Problems remained, however, many of them attributable to the political vagaries of funding and continuing difficulties with the application of the Rothschild principles and relations with the Medical Research Council. The names and dates of Chief Scientists from 1967 to 1990 are shown in Table 4.1.

Table 4.1   Chief Scientists 1967–1990

Time period	Chief Scientist
1967–1972	Dr R.H.L. (Dick) Cohen (also Deputy Chief Medical Officer)
1973–1977	Professor Sir Douglas Black
1978–1981	Professor Arthur Buller
1982–1985	Professor Sir Desmond Pond
1986–1990	Professor Francis O'Grady
1991–1997 (title changed to Director of Research and Development)	Professor Sir Michael Peckham

When Sir Douglas Black resigned from the post of Chief Scientist in 1977 there was some concern about his successor. The Research Unit Directors were keenly interested in this succession.[43] The Department of Health wanted to recruit an individual who had Medical Research Council relations and credentials. Two individuals – Professor A.C. Dornhorst (1915–2003) and Professor A. Buller (b. 1923) were about to retire from their membership of the Medical Research Council Clinical Research Board and were considered frontrunners for the post. Professor Dornhorst was Professor of Medicine at St George's Hospital Medical School. He was an outstanding clinician and a highly respected innovative scientist. He had been Reader in Medicine at St Thomas'. His major interests were in cardiovascular and respiratory medicine and he is credited with developing the concept of 'pink puffers' and 'blue bloaters' to distinguish different manifestations of chronic respiratory disease. Professor Buller, a highly regarded neurophysiologist, was Professor of Physiology at Bristol University, had worked in New Zealand with Professor Eccles (1903–1997) and had been a Senior Lecturer in Physiology at St Thomas'.

The Research Unit Directors Group met with Professor Abel Smith, who, at the time, was Special Adviser to the Secretary of State for Health, David Ennals (1922–1995), to express their interest in this crucial appointment. Abel Smith promised that he would discuss the Department's recommendations to the Secretary of State with the Directors, before briefing the former. The Unit Directors wanted to make sure that the individual appointed had direct NHS experience. Of the two favoured candidates, Dornhorst clearly had this. Buller, by contrast, was a basic scientist with little service experience. In his last years at St Thomas' Buller had spent some time with both the Professor of Medicine, Professor Sharpey-Schafer, and the Reader, Dr Dornhorst, on the Medical Unit as a titular Senior Registrar to gain some clinical experience.

In the event, Buller was appointed in 1978. Abel Smith confessed that he missed the relevant document in David Ennals' red box. It was slipped in at the bottom of a large pile of papers at a weekend, a common practice of civil servants wishing to obtain Secretary of State's approval without any interference! It was later stated that Buller had been chosen because he had administrative as well as scientific experience, having been Dean of the Medical School at Bristol. What the civil servants apparently did not appreciate was that, at that time, Deans at Bristol were elected for one year and it was customary for all Heads of Department to fulfil that role in turn!

Buller had two major concerns as Chief Scientist. He questioned the quality of much of the HSR commissioned by the Department of Health and the application of the Rothschild principles for the transfer of funds from the Medical Research Council to the Department. He was able to negotiate the return of the transferred funds to the Medical Research Council with a number of safeguards. These included the proviso that the Medical Research Council Board would have additional Department of Health representatives, would encourage HSR and would create a mechanism for its support. The terms of the agreement are detailed in the Department of Health's *Handbook of Research and Development*.[44]

Part of Buller's concern with the quality of HSR was influenced by his own background and training in the measurement of neurophysiological parameters and the suspicion that he, and many others, shared of the 'soft' findings and methods of social research. Some of this was justifiable. HSR, as a discipline, had developed relatively quickly and, as mentioned above, often in isolation from the assurance of quality from the parent disciplines. In addition, the Department of Health's commissions were not always couched in reasonable, specific terms and results were sometimes required for policy decisions far too rapidly to ensure that studies were adequately designed or executed.

Buller approached me shortly after he had been appointed to ask if I would help him and work as Deputy Chief Scientist for two or three days per week. I had already committed myself to spend six months on sabbatical in the US and in Europe, and I was unwilling to forgo this. So Professor Cole (1935–1988), with a background in the biological sciences, was appointed. I did, however, participate in and chair a number of the evaluations of HSR projects and units during this time.

This experience revealed the reality of some of Buller's concerns. His tenure as Chief Scientist was considered controversial by many HSR workers, particularly among the social scientists. He was not helped by the political turbulence and restriction of funds following the advent of a Conservative administration. Buller was succeeded as Chief Scientist in 1982 by Professor Sir Desmond Pond (1919–1986), Professor of Psychiatry at the London Hospital Medical School, who was more receptive to the importance of social science than his predecessor. He was also a peacemaker and his time as Chief Scientist was much less controversial.

The following anecdote might help to illustrate the confusion within the Department of Health about the nature of HSR. Dr Malcolm Godfrey (b. 1926), a Third Secretary of the Medical Research Council and later Dean of the Hammersmith Postgraduate Medical School, and I were invited, separately, to meet the Secretary of State for Health, Mr Patrick Jenkin (b. 1926). We were asked if we would like to be considered for the post of Chief Scientist to succeed Buller. I spent about 20 minutes with the Secretary of State. It was a pleasant meeting but I realised that he did not understand the difference in role and function of the Chief Scientist and the Department's Chief Scientific Officer – responsible for equipment, technical and scientific services, such as radiology or biochemistry. Malcolm Godfrey and I met subsequently to discuss how we should respond as we did not wish to compete against each other. After about two hours of discussion, we both concluded that neither of us wished to be considered for the post – we could not see how we could actually develop HSR in the prevailing political climate or how, as outsiders, we could influence the Department of Health to change its policies for research.

Sir Desmond Pond was succeeded in 1986 by Professor Francis O'Grady (b. 1925) who was Professor of Microbiology at the University of Nottingham and his time as Chief Scientist coincided with the House of Lords enquiry into Medical Research.[45] During O'Grady's tenure the amount of research carried out declined because of governmental restriction of resources and morale among researchers plummeted. His occupancy of the post is perhaps best remembered by his belief that the purpose of HSR was the support of Ministerial policies rather than the investigation and research into how the NHS could be made more effective and efficient. Perhaps the epitome of his reign was his valedictory statement that tried to reinterpret both the method and purpose of departmental support of HSR. I published a critique of O'Grady's stance and stout rebuttals of his views by Cohen and Godber, the originators of HSR, followed. It is worth considering the statement and responses in some detail to illuminate official thinking at this time.

Valedictory statement
In his valediction, O'Grady outlined his view of the history of HSR.[46] He considered that there was a great deal of confusion and states that there was:

> [a] belief, outside the Department, that its research exists to fund clinical research which is too close to service provision to command support from the MRC. This misunderstanding arises from the second confusion: the belief that the Department is responsible for the provision of services, and hence for the research necessary to advance it. It was plainly a surprise to the House of Lords Select Committee on Science and Technology in 1988 (perhaps, also, to the research community) to be told that the Department's research programme, like the Department itself, exists to support its Ministers in their policy development. However, while the programme itself is rooted in policy development, evidence of its usefulness is sought in improvements in the provision of services. It was this apparent dichotomy – in which those who can effect change in service provision do not define research needs, and those who define the research needs cannot directly effect the changes supported by the research – which led to the recommendation by the House of Lords Select Committee that a distinct effort should be made to ensure that the research needs of the NHS were addressed directly and separately from the policy research required by the Department of Health.
>
> The first main reason why the Department's research programme was not believed to be meeting its objectives, therefore, was that those objectives have been misunderstood. Its purpose was to support the need of policy development; but its critics claimed that it should have been supporting the clinical and operational needs of service provision.

Conflict

Apart from this confusion, conflict arose between the customers and contractors about the construction of the programme. Policy-makers find research useful when it illuminates and propels the policy development in hand. They need to turn in the relatively short term to agencies that will grasp what they are trying to do and provide quick and relevant responses. They are less likely to welcome agencies that want to debate the policy and its development, or the credibility of the proposals to advance it. Given the pressure of government business, they are also unlikely to want to devote much time to developing a long-term research strategy, or contemplating questions for the future, which are more likely to preoccupy their successors.

The views and needs of researchers are almost the exact converse. They do not want to be 'penny-in-the-slot' responders: they wish to participate in the policy debate, and they want to develop long-term plans to have time to speculate and innovate.

Whatever view is taken of the relative strengths of these positions, they plainly cannot coexist without modification. It is easy to say that the trick is to strike a balance that optimises the distribution of benefit. Failure to do so over a good many years has been the second major reason why the programme has been seen as less than a complete success from one or other side of the customer-contractor divide.

New Structure

These are, of course, not new revelations. Numerous attempts have been made over the years to get the balance right: to ensure that policy-makers were informed about research potential and their needs articulated in research terms; and to ensure that researchers acquired the skills and credibility which would enable them to respond efficiently to policy-makers' needs. The experiment in the 1970s with Research Liaison Groups (RLGs) was intended to provide the right kind of mix of policy-makers, research workers and research management to achieve the necessary interchange and planning. Some RLGs were very effective in tailoring proposals to the needs of their policy divisions. Their role was to advise the Department; but when they provided a coherent forward-plan, the forward spending pattern for research was inevitably fixed along established policy group lines. It became increasingly difficult to switch direction and, in particular, to deal with major, emerging cross-departmental issues.

A radical solution was adopted in 1986/87. Distribution of funding along established lines was swept away, and a high-level Departmental Research Committee redefined the Department's research needs in terms of priority themes for work that was currently engaging the Department's attention. This had the great advantage of focusing the programme into broad but defined areas, and excluding or relegating others. But the programme is still subject to the danger of self-perpetuation, constraining the development of new initiatives, as well as to creeping expansion – with a little ingenuity, customers are able to fit most of their preoccupations into the theme framework. The priority themes do not themselves amount to a research strategy. They simply identify a series of boundaries, and the programme is still in danger of remaining a differently packaged aggregate of discrete and disconnected policy needs.[46]

Responses to O'Grady

O'Grady's valediction went on to discuss relations with the Regions, the Medical Research Council and the Economic and Social Research Council and how difficult it was to develop a research strategy. It portrayed, however, a very singular view of HSR and its origins and governance and this led me to respond to it, partly to contradict some of the assertions about the views of the House of Lords.[47]

The valediction is a remarkably frank account of Professor O'Grady's views on DH-funded research. However, it gives a somewhat one-sided view of the development and present status of this research that needs to be countered by one of the individuals who has been involved in the process since the beginning. This is particularly necessary as Professor O'Grady expresses considerable disappointment when he considers the history of DHSS- (now D), funded research.

O'Grady does not clarify the cause of this disappointment but, from one of those involved in undertaking the sort of research he describes, similar expressions of dissatisfaction have come from the researchers' side as well over the years. To put this view into some sort of context, it is also important to discuss the evidence other than that produced by the Department of Health. Many of the issues that O'Grady discusses in his 'valediction' were drawn to the Department's attention by researchers some 20 years ago. It would indeed be unfortunate if Professor O'Grady's sense of disappointment were to be linked in the minds of readers exclusively with the faults of researchers!

Godber, the then Chief Medical Officer, in his preface to 'Portfolio for Health 1' gave a brief history of DHSS-supported research.[48] Stemming from initial interest, largely dominated by communicable disease and sanitary conditions, the Medical Research Council was established, leaving only a small research base at the Department. Godber then went on to describe how there was a resurgence in DHSS-funded research in the 1960s. However, Cohen, the first DHSS Chief Scientist, in the same volume,[48] described how only a minor element in the total research effort in the medical and allied social sciences is supported by the Department compared with the Medical Research Council.[38, p.18] As Cohen emphasised, an executive department cannot be considered in isolation from its place in the total administrative structure. Service research is a vital instrument for administrative planning and action. Its purpose is to help provide the framework within which service decisions are taken and evaluated. Such association needs to be close if those involved in research are to be alerted to problems of concern to those involved with service provision, and if administrators are to learn the appropriate uses and limitations of research which is 'like a pair of spectacles offering clearer and longer vision, and not like a magic wand to conjure up ready-made solutions and decisions.'

Cohen had already stated in 1971 that there was 'probably a need for an independent health services research council' because a government department is bound to be subject to the pressures of political and administrative expediencies which put the independence and continuity of its research policy and programme at risk. It would be unrealistic to deny that there is an inherent risk of this, and indeed it is right that there should be political interest in the priorities for government-financed research. The right equilibrium is a delicate one, and some form of machinery to protect this is probably necessary. It is also quite reasonably held that the quality and balance of a departmental research policy would be better assured and research more accountable if it were more open to independent scientific discussion, not only in retrospect, but also in the formative stage.

In his second report in 1973, Cohen was already demonstrating that the results of his improvements in structure were of benefit to both the Department and the NHS.[49] However, more recent publications have shown that these developments were not maintained over time.

The problems associated with DHSS-funded research over the years have been described in detail. Major concerns of the Nuffield Trust Research Unit Directors Group included the funding, approving and monitoring of the research and the need to provide a career in research. However, this meeting between individuals concerned with both the practice of research and its commissioning clearly demonstrated that a fruitful dialogue was possible.

This disquiet with the policies for health services research and its relevance to management were again expressed in a further Nuffield Trust publication.[43] It was evident from this that the authors considered that the plight of such research had not improved over the years, in spite of the lengthy debate and the recognition of its importance by a variety of eminent commentators – see, for example, Jennett [1926–2008] in his Rock Carling lecture.[50]

The major problem identified in the 1988 publication[45] was that the system supporting health services research had not succeeded in 'establishing a co-ordinated approach, and, despite sanguine hopes, the involvement of the actual customers of Health Services Research, the Regional and District Health Authorities, has diminished'. It goes on to say: 'Nevertheless, at a time when there is a greater need than ever before for Health Services Research, the mechanism for supporting and initiating research has become more bureaucratic and cumbersome and the impetus for research has faltered.'

This publication recognised that, with the advent of the Management Board and the new managerial structure in the NHS, a new opportunity was offered to ensure the effective application and undertaking of such research. It was also emphasised that such research is, by its very nature, long-term and multidisciplinary, and that it was essential to provide a stable and supportive environment if such research were to contribute to the development of long-term strategies and be sufficiently flexible to respond quickly to new situations. The Department of Health did not, however, choose to respond to this new opportunity.

O'Grady does not respond to this obvious sense of frustration by those involved in the research. He also suggests that there is some confusion between health services research and clinical research. He further asserts, wrongly in my view, that the Select Committee of the House of Lords was surprised to be told that the Department's research programme existed to support its Ministers in their policy development. It was precisely because the Committee saw that the Department operated its research programme exclusively in support of ministerial policy that it recommended steps to broaden the Department's research responsibilities. If one reads the House of Lords report 'Priorities in medical research' carefully, it should be evident that the Committee recognised the need for both research in support of Ministers and research in support of the National Health Service.[45] The committee was, however, surprised that in spite of the evident need for health services research and operational research to support the NHS, sufficient notice of these needs had not been taken by Ministers, the Department and others, nor had the necessary measures recommended to the Department and its Chief Scientists since the beginning of the 1970s been undertaken.

It was in view of this deficiency and the neglect by successive holders of the post of Chief Scientist that the Committee recommended the creation of a new body – a National Health Research Authority – and emphasised that distinct efforts should be made to support the research needs of the NHS. It noted how 'it is especially serious that so large an organisation as the NHS devotes so small a part of its budget to seeking how to improve its own operations.' The Committee emphasised the need to encourage the long-term development of public health and operational research by providing a flow of research contracts and career prospects capable of drawing talented researchers into the subject. They further recommended that, by creation of an appropriate body, first-class independent academic work attuned to the needs of the health service and the health departments would be provided.[47]

Sir George Godber also took exception to O'Grady's account.[51]

Walter Holland's commentary on Professor O'Grady's 'Valediction' is a valuable corrective, but there is more to be said. There were four Chief Scientists before O'Grady, not three, and the first of them, R.H.L Cohen, comments below on the 10-year period when he established and co-ordinated a rapidly growing programme of research before his year as Chief Scientist in 1972. The Chief Medical Officer's fund can be traced much farther back than the 1958 O'Grady mentions. For a century that fund had been used to meet the cost of small projects at the CMO's discretion – indeed, John Simon was given the same annual amount (£5000) as I inherited in 1960. There were, however, other departmental contributions for research and a larger commitment to some components of the NHS that made subsequent health service research practicable. At no time in my 34 years in the Department did I hear the view that we should not support research for the improvement of health care, but only for the advancement of ministerial policy. The advent of new knowledge must often shape policy rather than depend upon it.

The Public Health Laboratory Service (PHLS) was the largest early contribution in the NHS to a research system, even though its primary purpose was to support the control of communicable disease. The Emergency PHLS of wartime had already undertaken large-scale research into the efficacy of vaccines – first diphtheria, then pertussis – and had greatly improved the control of typhoid and paratyphoid by developing phage-typing of the causal organisms. Field trials of polio vaccine and validation of other vaccines followed during the 1950s and 1960s. The PHLS was the first element of the NHS to come into operation and was given early preference in capital allocation. Until the Board was established by law 10 years later, its administration was handled by the MRC but it always operated in close collaboration with the Ministry which funded it.

Good medical records in hospitals are essential for effective health services research, as for efficiency in hospital work. A working party chaired by Sir Ernest Rock Carling [1877–1960] and including such as John Ryle [1889–1950], Alan Moncrieff [1901–1971], Francis Avery Jones [1910–1998] and Percy Stocks [1889–1974] of the General Register Office (GRO) devised a standard summary form for the Hospital In-Patient Enquiry it proposed. Percy Stocks and I, as the group's amanuenses, planned the form not only for central analysis but as importantly to ensure better primary records. Most hospitals voluntarily adopted the forms to be completed for every tenth admission and in 1957 all were brought in. The GRO published annual studies that perhaps received more attention abroad than at home, but the greater gain was in general improvement of medical records and the use of the material by other researchers. Jerry Morris [1910–2009] was one of the first to take advantage of the material for a comparative study of surgical outcomes in different hospitals. Donald Acheson [1926–2009], with support from Nuffield, established the Oxford Record Linkage study for the purpose of outcome review. Later, Scotland was to develop this field faster and in greater detail. Logan at the GRO also developed morbidity studies in general practice in collaboration with the newly formed College.

Paul Lembcke [1908–1964] at Johns Hopkins had developed review of hospital activity in the United States that prompted similar study of lengths of stay in NHS hospitals by C. Donelan, reported to Senior Administrative Medical Officers (SAMOs) but not published, in the 1950s. Lloyd Hughes in the Liverpool Region and the King's Fund in London followed this up. Progressive reduction in stay made a rapid increase in turnover in acute beds possible, of the order of 50 per cent in the first decade of the NHS. The study at the Ministry and GRO by Brooke and Tooth of the even larger change in use of beds for the mentally ill led to a radical review of future provision for psychiatric illness. Various surgeons were developing short-stay programmes for some elective surgical procedures ranging from fenestration for otosclerosis to day surgery or injection methods for treatment of varicose veins. This last procedure, at the instance of J.O.F. Davies [1908–1978] when on secondment to the Ministry, was established in Manchester and at St Mary's on the system then used in Dublin, and was widely adopted thereafter with a great reduction in use of hospital beds and an increase in patients treated.

Much of this work was development rather than research, but it had to be fostered and often validated by modest research studies.

Mass screening by miniature radiography had been used in the control of pulmonary tuberculosis from the early days, but other screening procedures were being developed, using automated laboratory methods, for cervical cancer, phenylketonuria and hypothyroidism. Fortunately, we escaped the so-called multiphasic screening on which much was wasted elsewhere, and tonometry screening for glaucoma after a Ministry-sponsored study. J.M.G. Wilson played an important part in ensuring a balanced appraisal of these measures, and his report for the WHO is still an important resource document. Equally, Catherine Dennis kept us in close touch with the advances in and need for cardiac surgery and treatment of renal failure. The Standing Medical Advisory Committee was active in guiding policy, notably through Tom McKeown [1912–1988], Max Rosenheim [1908–1972] and Hedley Atkins [1905–1983].

A great deal of this kind of work was carried on in a rather disjointed way from the Department and there was close liaison with the MRC. The personal link with Harold Himsworth was close and stimulating, and in my own time the CMO's right to attend Council meetings was perhaps the most useful and informative privilege he had. That liaison led to the transfer of Dick Cohen in later 1962 to coordinate and develop the Ministry research work. Already the miniscule 'CMO's Fund' was overshadowed by special grants from reserve funds and it was obvious that much more was needed. That is for Dick Cohen himself to describe, but in my annual report for 1963 I could write: 'In the current financial year, £448 000 from specially allocated exchequer funds is being spent by hospital boards, and it is particularly encouraging that nearly half this effort is provided by Regional Boards.'

This superficial account cannot do justice to the very large effort made by the many members of the Standing Medical and other Advisory Committees, all heavily dependent on the background investigation and presentation by Ministry medical staff of which they made excellent use. One particular study was celebrated in its 42nd year by the Royal College of Obstetricians and Gynaecologists which suggested it and still participates fully. The Confidential Enquiry into Maternal Deaths must be one of the longest uninterrupted exercises in outcome and quality review. It may now be no more than a background to the more detailed evaluation of all obstetric and gynaecological work undertaken annually by such departments as that at St George's. But it was the forerunner of such as these and of perinatal death surveys, the recent studies of postoperative deaths and the Faculty of Anaesthetists' well-established surveys of deaths associated with anaesthesia, the first of which was organised 35 years ago.

A lot of this work seems crude by the standards we should apply today; perhaps it should have been more clearly envisaged and more rapidly developed. Nevertheless it was started and it began by intent – of people in the service, not of Ministers.'[51]

Dr Cohen, the first Chief Scientist joined the correspondence.[52]

It was plainly a surprise to the House of Lords Select Committee on Science and Technology, writes Professor O'Grady in his 'Valediction' to learn (if I understand him correctly) that the Department's research programme was not concerned directly with helping to meet the research needs of the NHS but existed solely for the development of ministerial policy. It is no wonder that they were surprised, for some of them must have known quite well that what they were being told was a travesty of the Department's historic responsibilities and powers. The Ministry of Health Act 1919 imposes on the Minister the duty to take all measures 'conducive to the health of the people including measures for the initiation and direction of research.' The National Health Service Act 1946 empowers him to 'conduct, or assist by grants or otherwise any other person to conduct, research into any matters relating to the causation, prevention, diagnosis or treatment of illness or mental defectiveness.' And the concordat between the Ministry and the Medical Research Council (MRC) in 1924, reaffirmed in 1949, which spells out their respective functions in some detail, lists among those of the former '… and to initiate and themselves direct research by such investigations as can best be carried out by the Ministry in the interests of public health administration, applied knowledge or medical services.' It is true that in the past the research needs of the Ministry had normally overlapped with the interests and responsibilities of the MRC so that initiation by reference to the MRC tended to be the most satisfactory procedure. But the Ministry's powers had never lapsed and clearly no further authority was needed for a more active role should changing circumstances make this necessary in order to fulfil its responsibilities.

The changed circumstance that led the Department to assume a new and major role was the recognition (which coincided, not altogether by chance, with George Godber becoming CMO) that, without large-scale service-related research and development, a comprehensive nation-wide service could not continue to function successfully for very much longer in the face of increasing public expectations and unprecedentedly rapid advances in science and technology. Thus in its origin and basis the primary purpose of the Department's research programme, as it was conceived and developed in the 1960s and well into the 1970s, was to support the provision and distribution of health and social care in the NHS; and it was by improvements in the NHS that the success of the programme was expected to be judged. If Ministers or Permanent Secretaries had thought that this was wrong and that they were being hijacked on a runaway train to an irrelevant and mistaken destination, I doubt if they would have encouraged expenditure on such research to grow from virtually nothing in 1960 to some £3 million 10 years later. Of course, we were also committed to research in relation to current ministerial policy and I do not deny that riding two horses which may not always be facing the same way can lead to complications (the possibility of conflict on these lines was the reason for the MRC being set up independently of the Ministry, to everyone's great advantage); I can only say that I never experienced even a hint of trouble myself in 11 years which included a change of government. But, in any case, is it seriously suggested, that, rather than run this risk, it would have been better to forgo the opportunity of setting in train support which the NHS badly needed and which no other source, local or central, was then in a position to provide, or probably has been since? As it happened, and we may have been lucky, Ministers seemed to welcome the idea of unbiased and free-ranging research as likely, given time, to help them in their policy decisions. I prefer this modest ambition of research-influenced policy to Professor O'Grady's more authoritarian alternative of 'policy-driven' research with the limitations on free enquiry and the veto on publication without ministerial approval to which it seems to have led.

In the early 1960s, when George Godber set us up in business, under his encouraging and watchful guiding eye, health services research was still a largely untested novelty. Hardly any work of the kind had been done in other countries and the few examples here were mainly some pioneering projects of high quality sponsored by the Nuffield Provincial Hospitals Trust under its then Secretary Gordon McLachlan, who was to become a friendly critic and collaborator and who elicited from us and published the two Portfolios for Health. We were fully prepared for our infant steps to be uncertain and progress slow. Right from the start, however, we found a reservoir of untapped goodwill towards practical work in support of the NHS and a readiness to take part by many experienced research workers including, among others, such people as Tom Whitehead, Archie Cochrane [1909–1988], Jerry Morris, Alan Williams, Richard Doll, Walter Holland, John Waterlow, Martin Roth, Margot Jefferys, Tom McKeown and George Knox. Much more quickly, therefore, than we had expected we were able to take the crucial step of setting up a framework of research units and other academic groups with broad terms of reference in agreed parts of the field. Equally vital was the willing collaboration of those involved in the actual day-to-day delivery of health care, including such SAMOs as J.O.F. Davis and John Revans [1911–1988], and many hospital doctors, GPs and nurses. This ensured that the research was likely to be genuinely relevant to service needs, that it could be carried out on site and, if successful, had a reasonable chance of being implemented. Initially, at least, we expected the main flow of ideas to be from the periphery to the centre rather than the other way round, but we looked forward to the traffic becoming increasingly two-way, to the mutual benefit of research workers and administrators and their education in each others' problems and ways of thought.

This is not the place for even a bird's eye view of the first 10 years. But by the end of that time we had set up a seemingly stable and adaptable base of research; we were making steady progress on a wide-ranging programme of good-quality work and were increasingly concentrating on themes of future priorities; we had given grants for several hundred spontaneously proposed individual projects; we had encouraged the recruitment and training of epidemiologists who were badly needed in the service and for whom there had been few openings; and, apart from research proper, we had used R&D funds and supervision to test and set up a substantial number of service and medical innovations which needed more controlled development or general-isation then was possible under the normal arrangements of local priorities. I think the record shows not only a good deal of solid benefit to the NHS but also that a lot of basic information was accumulated which should have been useful in forming or improving departmental policy decisions.

Unfortunately, as time went by, there was increasing cause for anxiety about the future. We had proved unable to provide the research staff with a long-term career structure offering reasonable security and prospects. The university departments which were the hosts for almost all the DHSS-financed units could not absorb permanently more than a very small proportion of the units' members. The Department itself was quite unsuitable as a home for academic staff whose future was in research and teaching. Some arrangement with the MRC would have been the best solution and very briefly seemed a future possibility when on their initiative, through Malcolm Godfrey, a joint unit was set up at Northwick Park; but no further progress was made.

Then out of the blue came Rothschild. But that is another story.'[52]

CONCLUSION

This chapter is based very much on my own experience and impressions. There is some overlap with Chapter 3 but it was considered important to repeat certain statements to provide a coherent picture. I hope it illustrates the many constraints and tensions in the development of HSR over the years. I felt it important to put on record how the vision (or lack of it) of previous Chief Scientists has had a crucial bearing on the research on which effective management of the NHS will always depend.

REFERENCES

1 Day, T.D. (1947). Membranous Nature of Interstitial Connective Tissue. *Lancet*, **250**, 945.
2 Day, T.D. (1948). Influence of Hydrogen Ions and Neutral Salts upon the Hydration of Interstitial Connective Tissue. *Nature*, **162**, 152–3.
3 Bradley, R.D., Gaskell, P., Holland, W.W., Lee, G. de J. and Young, I.M. (1954). The acid-base changes in arterial blood during adrenaline hyperpnoea in man. *Journal of Physiology*, **124**(2), 213–18.
4 Holland, W.W. and Young, I.M. (1956). Neonatal blood pressure in relation to maturity, mode of delivery, and condition at birth. *British Medical Journal*, **2**(5005), 1331–3.
5 Young, I.M. and Holland, W.W. (1958). Some physiological responses of neonatal arterial blood pressure and pulse rate. *British Medical Journal*, **34**(5091), 276–8.
6 Holland, W.W. and Young, I.M. (1958). *Neonatal Thermoregulation*. Montreal: International Paediatric Congress.
7 Holland, W.W. (1957). A clinical study of influenza in the Royal Air Force. *Lancet*, **273**(7000), 840–841.
8 Holland, W.W., Isaacs, A., Clarke, S.K. and Heath, R.D. (1958). A serological trial of asian-influenza vaccine after the autumn epidemics. *Lancet*, April: **1**(7025), 820–822.

9   McDonald, J.C., Wilson, J.S., Thorburn, W.B. and Holland, W.W. (1958). Acute respiratory disease in the RAF, 1955–1957. *British Medical Journal*, **2**(5098), 721–4.

10 Holland, W.W., McDonald, J.C. and Wilson, J.S. (1959). Asian Influenza in the Royal Air Force in the United Kingdom 1957–58. *Monthly Bulletin of the Ministry of Health and Public Health Laboratory Service*, **18**, 65–70.

11 Holland, W.W., Rowson, K.E.K., Taylor, C.E.D, Allan, A.B., French-Constant, M. and Smelt, C.M. (1960). Q fever in the RAF in Great Britain in 1958. *British Medical Journal*, **1**(5170), 387–90.

12 Holland, W.W., Tanner, E.I., Pereira, M.S. and Taylor, C.E.D. (1960). A study of the aetiology of respiratory disease in a general hospital. *British Medical Journal*, **1**(5190), 1917–22.

13 Holland, W.W., Colley, J.R. and Barraclough, M.A. (1960). Measurement of respiratory effort and assessment of a method of treating lower-respiratory-tract infections in small children. *Lancet*, **2**, 1166–7.

14 Holland, W.W. (1960). The treatment of the Nephrotic Syndrome in children. In: Milne, M.D. (ed.), *Recent Advances in Renal Disease*, London: Royal College of Physicians, Pitman Medical Publishing, p. 123.

15 Holland, W.W., Doll, R. and Carter, C.O. (1962). The mortality from leukaemia and other cancers among patients with Down's syndrome and among their parents. *British Journal of Cancer*, **16**, 177–86.

16 Holland, W.W. (1964). *Epidemiological Surveys of Chronic Respiratory Disease in England*. MD Thesis, University of London.

17 Holland, W.W. and Reid, D.D. (1965). The urban factor in chronic bronchitis. *Lancet*, **1**, 445–8.

18 Holland, W.W. and Wolff, H.S. (1961). Blood pressure measurement without observer variability. *Journal of Physiology*, **1569**(2).

19 Holland, W.W. (1962). The reduction of observer variability in the measurement of blood pressure. In: Pemberton, J. (ed), *Epidemiology: Reports on Research and Teaching, 1962–1963*. Oxford: Oxford University Press.

20 Holland, W.W. and Humerfelt, S. (1964). Measurement of blood pressure. Comparison of intra-arterial and cuff values. *British Medical Journal*, **2**, 1241–3.

21 Holland, W.W., Reid, D.D., Seltser, R. and Stone, R.W. (1965). Respiratory disease in England and the United States. Studies of comparative prevalence. *Archives of Environmental Health*, **10**, 338–43.

22 Stone, R.W. and Holland, W.W. (1965). Respiratory disorders in United States East Coast Telephone area. *American Journal of Epidemiology*, **82**, 92–101.

23 Holland, W.W., Reid, D.D., Humerfelt, S. and Rose, G. (1966). A cardiovascular survey of British postal workers. *Lancet*, **1**, 614–18.

24 Reid, D.D., Holland, W.W. and Rose, G.A. (1967). An Anglo-American cardiovascular comparison. *Lancet*, **2**, 1357–78.

25 Holland, W.W., De Bono, E. and Goldman, A.J. (1964). Inpatient records: an investigation of their content and handling at St Thomas' Hospital. *Lancet*, **1**, 819–21.

26 Holland, W.W. (1965). Experiments in the development of data processing systems for medical records. In: *Mathematics and Computer Science in Biology and Medicine*. London: Medical Research Council, pp. 11–21.

27 Colley, J.R. and Holland, W.W. (1967). Social and environmental factors in respiratory disease: a preliminary report. *Archives of Environmental Health*, **14**, 157–61.

28 Holland, W.W., Halil, T., Bennett, A.E. and Elliott, A. (1969). Indications for measures to be taken in childhood to prevent chronic respiratory disease. *Milbank Memorial Fund Quarterly*, **47**(3), Part 2, 215–27.

29 Holland, W.W., Kasap, H.S., Colley, J.R. and Cormack, W. (1969). Respiratory symptoms and ventilatory function: a family study. *British Journal of Preventive and Social Medicine*, **23**, 77–84.

30 Colley, J.R., Holland, W.W. and Corkhill, R.T. (1974). Influence of passive smoking and parental phlegm on pneumonia and bronchitis in early childhood. *Lancet*, **2**, 1031–4.

31 Leeder, S.R., Corkhill, R.T., Irwig, L.M., Holland, W.W. and Colley, J.R. (1976). Influence of family factors on the incidence of lower respiratory illness during the first year of life. *British Journal of Preventive and Social Medicine*, **30**, 203–12.

32 Leeder, S.R., Corkhill, R.T., Wysocki, M.J. and Holland, W.W. (1976). Influence of personal and family factors on ventilatory function of children. *British Journal of Preventive and Social Medicine*, **30**, 219–24.

33 Colley, J.R., Holland, W.W., Leeder, S.R. and Corkhill, R.T. (1976). Respiratory function of infants in relation to subsequent respiratory disease: an epidemiological study. *Bulletin Physiologie, Pathologie, Respiratoire*, **12**, 651–7.

34 Holland, W.W. and Elliott, A. (1968). Cigarette smoking, respiratory symptoms and anti-smoking propaganda. An experiment. *Lancet*, **1**, 41–3.

35 Holland, W.W., Halil ,T., Bennett, A.E. and Elliott, A. (1969). Factors influencing the onset of chronic respiratory disease. *British Medical Journal*, **2**, 205–8.

36 Bland, J.M., Holland, W.W. and Elliott, A. (1974). The development of respiratory symptoms in a cohort of Kent school children. *Bulletin Physiologie, Pathologie, Respiratoire*, **10**, 699–715.

37 Landsborough Thomson, A. (1975). *Half a Century of Medical Research. Volume 1 Origins and Policies of the MRC (UK). Volume 2 The Programme of the MRC (UK)*. London: HMSO.

38 Holland, W.W. (2002). *Foundations for Health Improvement. Productive Epidemiological Public Health Research 1919–1998*. London: The Nuffield Trust, The Stationery Office.

39 McLachlan, G.A. (1992). *History of the Nuffield Provincial Hospitals Trust*. London: Nuffield Provincial Hospitals Trust.

40 Munk's Roll (2008). London: Royal College of Physicians.

41 Rothschild Report (1971). The organisation and management of Government R&D. In: *Cabinet Office: A Framework for Government Research and Development*. London: HMSO.

42   Kogan, M., Korman, N. and Henkel, M. (1980). *Government Commissioning of Research: A Case Study.* London: Department of Government, Brunel University.
43   McLachlan, G.A. (ed.) (1978). *Five Years After. A Review of Health Care Research Management After Rothschild.* Oxford: Oxford University Press for the Nuffield Provincial Hospitals Trust.
44   Department of Health (1981). *Handbook of Research and Development.* London: HMSO, Appendix 3, pp. 8–13.
45   Report of the House of Lords Sub-Committee of the Select Committee on Science and Technology (1988). *Priorities in Medical Research .* London: HMSO.
46   O'Grady, F. (1990). *Valediction. A Personal View from Professor Francis O'Grady, Chief Scientist of the Department of Health, 1986–1990.* Department of Health Yearbook of Research and Development. London: HMSO, pp. 1–5.
47   Holland, W.W. (1991). Personal view on valediction. *Journal of Public Health Medicine*, **13**, 344–8 (by permission of Oxford University Press).
48   McLachlan, G.A. (ed.) (1971). *Portfolio for Health 1. The Role and Programme of the DHSS in Health Services Research. Problems and Progress in Medical Care. 6th Series. Essays on Current Research.* London: Oxford University Press for the Nuffield Provincial Hospitals Trust, pp. xii–xiv.
49   McLachlan, G.A. (ed.) (1973). *Portfolio for Health 2. The Developing Programme of the DHSS in Health Services Research. Problems and Progress in Medical Care. 8th Series. Essays on Current Research.* London: Oxford University Press for the Nuffield Provincial Hospitals Trust.
50   Jennett, B. (1984). *High Technology Medicine. Benefits and Burdens. Rock Carling Fellowship, 1983.* London: Nuffield Provincial Hospitals Trust.
51   Godber, G.E. (1992). The Health Department and research. *Journal of Public Health Medicine*, **14**, 339–41.
52   Cohen, R.H.L. (1992). The Health Department and research. *Journal of Public Health Medicine*, **14**, 341–2.

APPENDIX

Key institutions in the US visited in 1961–1962

University of Maryland Medical School, Maryland
Harvard University Medical School, Boston
Harvard University School of Public Health, Boston
Boston University Medical School, Boston
Chicago University Medical School, Chicago
Illinois University Medical School, Chicago
University of California School of Public Health, Berkeley
University of California School of Medicine, San Francisco
University of California School of Medicine and Public Health, Los Angeles

School of Medicine, Cincinnati
School of Medicine, University of Colorado, Denver
School of Medicine, University of Alabama, Birmingham
School of Public Health, University of Michigan, Ann Arbor
School of Public Health and Medicine, University of North Carolina, Chapel Hill
Columbia School of Public Health, New York
School of Medicine, State University of New York, Brooklyn
School of Medicine, University of Buffalo, New York

5. Organisational and funding issues

ORGANISATION

HSR, in contrast to much laboratory research, is usually complex, takes a considerable amount of time to plan and to carry out, and requires a great deal of competent organisation to ensure the involvement and commitment of those responsible for implementing any findings. For such research to be successful, therefore, it needs to have a stable, long-term base. The cooperation of several disciplines in its design and execution is also essential.

In theory, multidisciplinary working is an attractive concept; in practice it presents many difficulties and requires individuals of the highest ability and motivation. And there are few, if any, specific training courses available, despite the fact that methods in research techniques are now taught at Masters level.

Multidisciplinarity

HSR involves medically qualified individuals, statisticians, social scientists – such as sociologists, psychologists and economists – and will sometimes also require the expertise of management science and operational research. The research unit on Social Medicine and Health Services Research at St Thomas' Hospital Medical School, which was set up in 1967, was one of the first multidisciplinary units to be established in the UK and has provided a model for subsequent multidisciplinary working.

A central problem in this area of work is that of academic commitment and advancement. Individuals who wish to pursue an academic career are recognised by their contribution to their parent subject. Social scientists undertaking HSR in a multidisciplinary unit, for example, require recognition as credible sociologists or psychologists within their own discipline. Their expertise and acknowledgement for future careers must come not only from the HSR community, but largely and mainly from their own specialty. The same is true for the other disciplines. The quality of the contribution of each of the relevant disciplines involved in a particular investigation must be of a high standard and recognised as such by their peers as well as the wider research team.

Another potential problem that can arise in multidisciplinary research is the necessity to focus on the original and central objectives of a particular project without being sidetracked into other interesting lines of investigation, relevant perhaps to only one of the disciplines involved. Our research on disability is a good example of this.

The main question the research needed to answer was the frequency of different forms of disability and their progression. The social scientists were concerned both with methods of classification of disability and with the social effects of different grades of disability. The medical researchers were more focused on the aetiology of different forms of disability as well as their effects on daily living. All these questions were important and relevant but the central problem was how many people were disabled, what grades of severity were identified and what services needed to be provided.[1] *The National Study of Health and Growth* was another example of how the multidisciplinary team needed to concentrate on the central issue – did children in different ethnic groups, social circumstances and levels of deprivation differ in changes in their height and weight, since this might indicate that the withdrawal of free school milk and meals was having a measurable effect of the health of primary school children? The statisticians involved in the study could have been more concerned with the development of statistical measures to identify changes in height or weight or the measurement of rates of growth rather than in simple identification of changes in height or weight in different groups. Such simple and reliable measures were likely to be of far greater significance to policy-makers than sophisticated mathematical models. Similarly, the medical members of the team needed to focus on the development of methods to chart changes in health over time rather than the relationship of physical health conditions to changes in height or weight. The latter was of course important but not central to the fundamental research question of whether changes in social and environmental circumstances (such as withdrawal of free school meals and milk) were related to health and nutrition.[2] There is also a real need for good communication between those who plan a particular project and those who actually carry out the research. They frequently have insufficient contact since most health services and epidemiological research involves the use of ancillary staff, such as fieldworkers, in the collection of data.

The St Thomas' Unit

As noted above, the Unit at St Thomas' Hospital Medical School provided the first model for the organisation of such multidisciplinary work.

The research unit was organised into three main divisions:

- Medicine – subdivided into epidemiology, medical care and general practice;
- Social science, including sociology, psychology and economics; and
- Statistics.

Each member of the department was identified by the nature of their qualifications with one of these divisions. Each separate discipline within a division was led by a senior colleague. Thus, in the Medical Division there was a lead epidemiologist, a lead physician and a lead general practitioner and the same applied in the Social Science Division.

Each lead individual had two main responsibilities. They had, first, to provide the necessary specialist input to the research being undertaken and, second, to ensure its quality. Each project had an individual who assumed an overall leadership role in its initiation, design and execution. The research team consisted of individuals from all the disciplines required and members of the team were accountable for their activities to the project leader. Project leaders had authority over the conduct of their projects and usually oversaw a number of fieldworkers and research assistants. As well as being accountable to their project leader, the team members reported to the head of their own discipline who was responsible for training and for maintaining and advancing the standards of that specialty. These lead specialists were also responsible for the effectiveness of the relevant discipline and the professional competence and well-being of the individuals within it and thus the Unit worked to control and advance research in a truly multidisciplinary way.

The Statistical Division stood slightly apart. Although central in its role within the Unit and its research activities, it was organised more as a service section. Its members were accountable to the head statistician for the quality of statistical work and to their project leader for their specific activities. Of course, this form of structure required a great deal of coordination since every research project required the participation of a senior statistician and several assistants.

In the selection and execution of multidisciplinary research, there has to be an effective central coordinating mechanism that decides on priorities. In our case, the Head and Deputy Head of the Department were accountable for all the research being undertaken. The Head of Department had to ensure that decisions on priorities, methods, choice of subjects and other relevant matters were taken with the full cooperation and commitment of the heads of all the disciplines so that the research was of acceptable quality.

The effectiveness of a research unit is judged by its results and one of the most important contributions to be made by multidisciplinary working lies not only in the production of useful research findings but also in education and in the transmission of ideas.

The effectiveness of our research can be illustrated by the influence of our studies in multiphasic screening in the NHS,[3] *The National Study of Health and Growth*, on government policy on the provision of free school milk and meals for primary school children,[2] and the studies on factors influencing school children to take up smoking cigarettes.[4]

These studies were important in the education of both health service managers and public health practitioners in demonstrating how and why measures of health care need were important and what methods could be used. The ideas developed by health service researchers have been widely disseminated and are now accepted as 'evidence-based medicine'.

The physical location of such research units is important. A site within an institution, such as a Medical School, with close links to clinical practice, produces a number of undoubted benefits which are difficult to quantify. The continual cooperation of statisticians, social scientists and doctors within the St Thomas' Unit, for example, undoubtedly broadened the outlook and education of all three disciplines. The existence of the Unit also had an influence on the staff of the Hospital and Medical School and played and continues to play a role in policy-making and in the education of people working within the institution as a whole. It is vital that research, particularly applied research, of this type is not separated from service and education.

FUNDING

In the 1960s there were four major sources of funds for medical research.

The Medical Research Council

The first and most prestigious of these sources was the Medical Research Council, the origin of which has already been described. The Medical Research Council has a procedure of peer review for consideration of grant proposals. In general the Medical Research Council funded basic research and was not particularly sympathetic to applied or clinical research – as reflected by the membership of its Council and Grant Committees. Although funds were disbursed for epidemiological work, most of this was concerned with the causes and mechanisms of diseases.

The history of the role of the Medical Research Council in the development of research in the UK is very distinguished. The organisation was created before the First World War partly because of problems with tuberculosis and the appreciation that to cope with this disease research was needed.

During the First World War the nascent Medical Research Council played an important role in research on such problems as the prevention and treatment of 'trench foot', a serious problem among soldiers serving in the trenches in France. After the war, the organisation expanded and established both a central research facility, the National Institute of Medical Research, as well as a number of research units tackling specific medical problems – for example, nutrition – as well as supporting investigator-initiated research proposals. In view of the thorough historical analysis of the Medical Research Council by Landsborough Thomson[5] I will not invade this territory, except to highlight certain characteristics, some of which were copied for later application by the Department of Health.

Training

Throughout its existence the Medical Research Council has recognised that in order to develop good medical health research the individuals involved require training. The universities had an obvious function in provision of the bulk of training, but as an independent research body, the Medical Research Council could and did provide additional resources both to fill gaps and complement the facilities of the universities. This was by the establishment of research fellowships at both junior and senior level for individuals who wished to pursue research, and which enabled the fellows to work in a Medical Research Council Research Unit, a university department or to obtain experience overseas, for example in the US. Some of these overseas fellowships were funded by charitable foundations, for example Rockefeller, and administered by the Medical Research Council. Many of the leaders of Medicine in the UK have benefited from holding one or other research training fellowships.

Research

The major strength of the Medical Research Council has always been its research support. It has achieved this by requesting applications from researchers in specific areas, general subjects and the development of methodology. In addition, in areas where a special need has been identified, research units have been created. These have, in almost every case, been closed down after the retirement or death of their Director – as, for example, with the closure of the Epidemiological Research Unit in Cardiff directed by Archie Cochrane, and the Social Medicine Research Unit at the London Hospital directed by Jerry Morris. The research supported has largely been in basic subjects such as biochemistry, physiology or genetics. But the Medical Research Council has also supported research on specific applications or diseases such as pneumoconiosis and cardiovascular disease. As Landsborough Thomson admits, however, there has been a reluctance to support research on preventive medicine because of the 'difficulty of application'.[5]

Advice

At all times the Medical Research Council has had working groups or committees which have advised government, the Medical Research Council and the NHS on specific topics – for example, influenza immunisation, infection in hospitals and diet. These bodies functioned both as sources of advice on health policy as well as on areas requiring research development. The Medical Research Council has supported certain activities, such as medical statistics and biological standards, requiring specific expertise or a critical mass of experts. At one stage it also administered the PHLS.

The record of the Medical Research Council in fulfilling its research function has been exemplified both by the results of individual pieces of research, such as those on penicillin, cancer of the lung and coronary heart disease, but also by the outstanding number of Nobel Laureates and other internationally recognised distinctions of the researchers it has supported. Most of the individuals who have been supported by the Medical Research Council regard it with respect and gratitude as well as admiration. Most accept that the decisions, for example in the highly competitive field of research grant applications, have been fair. It has maintained an enviable level of control of the quality of research it supports through its periodic reviews of units, programme grants and so on. The model and methods of research prioritisation, project selection, and assessment both of projects and individuals are universally admired, copied and considered as a model of the conduct of a research body.

Nonetheless it must be accepted that there are some criticisms of Medical Research Council activities. The resources for research are always limited and only a very small proportion of applications for research support are funded. Thus a major hindrance has always been a lack of funds. But as most decisions are made by scientists the decisions are often blinkered and dependent on the disciplinary knowledge, prejudices and experience of those in positions of authority within the organisation and its advisory committees. This has meant that, in the view of many, money is spent, for example, on numerous complex genetic, molecular investigations with relatively little on the more mundane problems of, for example, the treatment of infections in general practice. This concentration on basic science led to the criticism of the Research Councils by Lord Rothschild and his Central Policy Review Staff and to the changes recounted above.[6]

The Medical Research Council had three major research units whose interest was in epidemiology. The Social Medicine Research Unit, under the directorship of Professor Jerry Morris, was largely concerned with coronary heart disease at the London Hospital Medical School. The Statistical Research Unit under the leadership of Professor Sir Austin Bradford Hill and later Dr Richard Doll at the LSHTM was mainly interested in cancer of the lung and in developing and advising on statistical methods. The Epidemiological Research Unit under Professor Archie Cochrane in Cardiff – an offshoot of the Pneumoconiosis Research Unit led by Professor J. Gilson – was concerned with general epidemiology particularly in pulmonary and other chronic diseases.

Locally Organised Clinical Research

The second source of funds was from what was known as Locally Organised Clinical Research (LOCR), disbursed by Regional Committees from NHS resources. Grants from this source were usually given for identifiable short-term clinical projects. Applications were subjected to a review process but this was not as rigorous as that of the Medical Research Council.

Medical Charities

The third source of funding came from medical charities, such as the Imperial Cancer Research Fund and the Chest Heart and Stroke Association. These grants were also subject to a reasonably rigorous review process and were limited to the disease of interest to the individual charity.

Hospital Endowment Funds

The fourth source was the Endowment Funds of individual hospitals. The Endowment Funds were the residual funds of the voluntary hospitals which remained under their jurisdiction after the creation of the NHS. Their size depended on the wealth of the individual hospital in 1948. The funds of St Bartholomew's Hospital and St Thomas' Hospital, two of the oldest hospital institutions founded in the eleventh and twelfth centuries respectively, were, therefore, very substantial. In addition to the original sum available (several tens of millions of pounds), these hospitals had Boards of Governors, usually made up of eminent individuals well-versed in finance, who ensured that the funds were invested profitably. The income from the Endowment Funds was used by the institutions to improve the conditions of staff and patients – for example, by providing library services, training catering staff, owning and managing nurses' residences. Most of the hospitals also used a small proportion of the income from the funds for clinical research considered important for improvement of patient care. Review of the research proposals was not as rigorous as for any of the other research funding organisations and depended largely on whether particular individuals or proposals were of interest to the senior members of the staff of the hospital.

Department of Health

There was no specific research funding source for HSR. Almost all HSR before and in the early 1960s was undertaken by a small, in-house, research unit in the Ministry of Health. The few Ministry officials doing this type of research were either social scientists or statisticians. With the appointment of Sir George Godber as Chief Medical Officer, questions on health services, their function and performance, were beginning to be asked. The Medical Division of the Ministry had a Principal (a middle grade civil servant, John Cornish) who had worked in Operational Research (OR) during the Second World War. He recognised the need for HSR which he considered to be a form of OR. Godber had also recruited two medical officers with a background in research whose work and influence have been described earlier (see Chapter 3) – Dr R.H.L. (Dick) Cohen, who had been a Deputy Secretary of the Medical Research Council and Dr J.M.G. (Max) Wilson.

Table 5.1   Research Funding by the Department of Health

1964/65	Clinical	40 000		(272 000)
	Operational	100 000	240 000	(681 000)
	Equipment, Building	100 000	(1 634 000)	(681 000)
	Decentralised	400 000 (LOCR)		(2 724 000)
1967/68	Total 1 750 000 including computers			(10 789 00)
1970/71	Total 5 620 000 including LOCR 940 000			(29 771 000)
1971/72	Total Research 5 500 000 of which LOCR = 930 000			(28 229 000)
1972/73	Total Research 6 915 000 of which LOCR = 1 113 000			(33 413 000)
1973/74	Estimated Total Research 11 705 000 of which LOCR = 1 750 000			(50 937 000)
1977/78	Health Services	4 134 000		(13 603 000)
	Personal Social Services	2 887 000		(9 500 000)
	Other (including social security, computers, building, MRC, LOCR)	13 722 000		(45 152 000)
	Total	20 743 000		(68 255 000)
1978/79	Health Services	4 364 000		(12 896 000)
	Personal Social Services	3 456 000		(10 213 000)
	Other	14 177 000		(41 894 000)
	Total	21 997 000		(65 003 000)
1979/80	Health Services	4 865 000		(12 667 000)
	Personal Social Services	4 246 000		(11 055 000)
	Other	15 972 000		(41 585 000)
	Total	25 083 000		(65 307 000)
1980/81	Health Services	5 784 000		(13 651 000)
	Personal Social Services	5 323 000		(12 563 000)
	Other	19 646 000		(46 368 000)
	Total	30 756 000		(72 582 000)
1981/82	Total	22 831 000		(50 758 000)
	(HPSS/SS)	13 842 000		(30 774 000)
1982/83	Total	22 681 000		(48 855 000)
	(HPSS/SS)	13 140 000		(28 304 000)
1983/84	Total	19 361 000		(39 978 000)
	(HPSS/SS)	11 534 000		(23 816 000)

Table 5.1 Continued

1984/85	Total	18 584 000	(37 054 000)
	(HPSS/SS)	11 147 000	(22 226 000)
1985/86	Total	20 456 000	(40 456 000)
	(HPSS/SS)	11 351 000	(22 219 000)
1986/87	Total	23 195 000	(43 805 000)
	(HPSS/SS)	12 664 000	(23 917 000)
1987/88	Total	25 904 000	(46 978 000)
	(HPSS/SS)	14 614 000	(26 503 000)

Note: Values in 2009 in brackets. HPSS/SS: Health and Personal Social Services/Social Security.

Table 5.2   Research expenditure for selected units

	St Thomas'	Newcastle	Birmingham/Whitehead
1970	(608 000)	(94 000)	(816 000)
	110 000	17 000	147 500
1971/72	(641 000)	(170 000)	(848 000)
	121 000	32 000	160 000
1978/79	(845 000)	(312 000)	(671 000)
	285 800	105 600	227 226
1980/81	(751 000)	(366 000)	(1 093 000)
	318 000	155 200	462 900
1981/82	(900 000)	(427 000)	(1 023 000)
	405 000	192 000	460 000
1982/83	(1 191 000)	(554 000)	(1 299 000)
	552 700	257 400	603 000
1983/84	(1 242 000)	(800 000)	(1 192 000)
	601 500	387 400	577 200
1984/85	(1 092 000)	(1 002 000)	(1 235 000)
	547 900	502 500	619 300
1985/86	(1 119 000)	(936 000)	(1 067 000)
	571 500	478 000	545 000
1986/87	(834 000)	(1 032 000)	(1 185 000)
	441 700	546 300	627 400
1987/88	(1 502 000)	(981 000)	(519 000)
	828 000	540 900	286 300
1989/90	(1 439 000)	(815 000)	(1 105 000)
	876 671	496 673	673 351

Note: Values in 2009 in brackets.

Table 5.1 shows the expenditure by the Department of Health between 1964/65 and 1987/88. Two figures are given – the actual amount spent and the equivalent value in 2009 (in brackets). The amount spent increased rapidly in the period 1964–1973, slowed or diminished between 1977/78 and 1979/80, concomitant with the problems in the UK economy, increased by a small amount until 1982, diminished until 1985 when it again began to increase but by only a small amount.

To examine the changes in funding for units, three illustrative examples are shown in Table 5.2: St Thomas', a general purpose relatively large unit; Newcastle, another general purpose unit outside London; and Professor Whitehead's unit in Birmingham which was largely involved in research on laboratory medicine, particularly chemical pathology. All three units started at a relatively low level. Although there were fluctuations over the period 1970 to 1989/90, to some extent coincidental with the total research expenditures shown in Table 5.1, growth was relatively constant. The funding for St Thomas' more than doubled (in 2009 terms) over the period. Birmingham, starting at a higher level, had an increase of almost 50 per cent over the period. Newcastle, starting at a much lower level, increased its funding almost eightfold. Examination of the funding of these units, rather than the total expenditure by the Department of Health, illustrates the consistency of support by the Department of Health for research units. The brunt of reductions in expenditure in times of shortages and of increases in times of plenty was, therefore, borne by variation in grants for individual projects. Research Units were accepted by the Department of Health as an essential element in HSR. At times when the Department had its revenue funding limited for economic and political reasons, therefore, the Research Units were still able to retain their core funding in contrast to project funds available to all researchers.

Of course the sums listed for the three units are not necessarily the total amount spent on research in these centres. Each of them sought and attracted funding from other sources, including charities, industry, or international donors such as the World Health Organisation and the European Community as well as additional project funding from the Department of Health. These funds helped to cushion the year-on-year variations in funding in order to maintain stability for unit staff.

ACKNOWLEDGEMENT

Dr Saka Omer of the National Audit Office was kind enough to provide the data that enabled the conversion of expenditure over time to 2009 values.

REFERENCES

1 Bennett, A.E., Garrod, J. and Halil, T. (1970). Chronic disease and disability in the community: a prevalence study. *British Medical Journal*, **2**, 762–4.
2 Rona, R.J., Chinn, S. (1999). *The National Study of Health and Growth*. London: Oxford University Press.
3 South East London Screening Study Group (1977). A controlled trial of multiphasic screening in middle-age: results of the South East London Screening Study. *International Journal of Epidemiology*, **6**, 357–63.
4 Bewley, B.R., Bland, J.M. and Harris, R. (1974). Factors associated with the starting of cigarette smoking in primary school children. *British Journal of Preventive and Social Medicine*, **28**, 37–44.
5 Landsborough Thomson, A. (1978). *Half a Century of Medical Research. A Comprehensive History of the MRC*. London: HMSO.
6 Rothschild Report (1971). The organisation and management of Government R&D. In: *Cabinet Office: A Framework for Government Research and Development*. London: HMSO.

6. Health services research in practice

INTRODUCTION

In its early years, the Department of Health had begun to become interested in planning new health services as well as altering old ones. In practice, planning can either be based on intuition, prior experience and knowledge or on the development of models which can be used to predict likely outcomes. The setting of priorities, for any activity, is difficult. It can be based on beliefs or better on actual evidence – but their acceptance may be problematic if they differ from the hopes and beliefs of those responsible for their implementation. If the full promise of this kind of research is to be realised, then it has to tackle difficult problems and the clear goal at this time was to develop a model that would enable the Department to plan for the total need of care as well as for individual aspects and to carry out effective evaluation. Although important advances were being made in the studies of need, the holistic planning for health services remained a very complex problem although it was the ultimate objective. This type of planning development was advocated particularly by the Department's Operational Research Branch which was staffed by highly competent researchers with experience in operational research from the Second World War.

Operational research had been extremely influential and successful in the planning of services for local government. The operational researchers themselves, however, did not fully appreciate the difference between local government and the NHS and the complexities of planning a service involving many different providers and professions in many locations. This is in stark contrast with the planning of some more focused local government services such as, for example, waste disposal. The Department of Health had commissioned the Operational Research Branch to develop a global model for the provision of health services, and this was considered very influential by some of its senior officials. There were others responsible for various NHS decisions, however, who were somewhat more dubious about the methods and conclusions of operational research. In the light of this, the Department of Health set up an independent review chaired by Sir Douglas Black and included the

Professor of Management Science from the University of Warwick and myself. We took evidence from a large number of the deputy and under-secretaries who were responsible for different aspects of the Department of Health and of the NHS.

One fascinating meeting brought all these individuals together to present their views to us. I have never, before or since, observed such skilful stiletto and rapier play in any meeting and it demonstrated the divisions that existed in the interpretation and usefulness of the model developed by the Operational Research Division. It may have been, at least in part, this meeting that persuaded the Black Committee to advise the Department of Health that, while operational research was extremely helpful in solving individual problems in the health service, it could not be used effectively in the development of a holistic model of the NHS. As a result, it was agreed that more specific questions needed to be asked and more research had to be done on both the development and the evaluation of individual health services.

DEVELOPMENT AND EVALUATION OF NEW WAYS OF PROVIDING HEALTH SERVICES

In a new departure, the Department of Health thus began to consider alternative ways of providing services and to develop promising ideas on a trial basis and subject them to scientifically sound evaluation. Previously, policy had always been decided by the Department on the basis of value judgement and experience rather than as a result of rigorous evaluation and scientific experimentation. Even so, health policy research was still viewed with some suspicion and was not universally accepted or adopted. An example of this was when the Department of Health decided to begin to build new hospitals and to explore alternative models rather than follow previous practice. Because of the advances in health care, many conditions that had previously been subject to inpatient care were considered to be candidates for care within the community. Thus the new hospitals were to be designed so that community care could be maximised with more outpatient and diagnostic facilities and fewer inpatient beds. Two prototype hospitals were to be built, one at Frimley and one at Bury St Edmunds; and the St Thomas' Research Unit was invited to put forward proposals for the evaluation of the Frimley Hospital.

The Unit proposed to use a number of indicator conditions to test whether the change from inpatient to community care could be implemented and what its costs and consequences would be. The Unit put forward four areas for study. The first was psychiatric care. There was already a large psychiatric hospital near Basingstoke, Hampshire with about 1400 inpatients and we wanted to see whether they could be discharged successfully into the community.[1, 2] Second, we proposed an experiment on short-stay surgery by randomising individuals for operations for hernia and varicose veins to a stay of two days rather than the standard seven to ten days.[3] Third, we investigated the use that could be made of general practitioners taking responsibility for inpatients.[4] Finally, we looked at type of care by developing a follow up study for a chronic condition – stroke – by identifying all cases that occurred within the geographical area of Frimley and following them up until they died or for four years.[5] I do not intend to deal with the actual experiments that we did at this time except to describe the decision-making process for the commissioning of this research which illustrated the problems that researchers had with the Department of Health.

The meeting to decide whether the St Thomas' Unit should undertake this research, held in 1968, was attended by several senior members of the Department, as well as by the Chief Scientist, Dr R.H.L. (Dick) Cohen. After our presentation, however, a very senior official queried whether research commissioned by the Department of Health could actually question policy that had been adopted by Ministers. The Unit, as well as the Chief Scientist, stated that one of the purposes of research was to question policy; it would be pointless if its sole purpose was to endorse any policy that had been decided. Furthermore, policy at one time is not necessarily right for the future and the whole function of research was to question. The Department maintained its stance and refused, at the meeting, to sanction that the research be started. This was deferred for consideration by Ministers and it took approximately six months for the decision to be reached that the position taken by the research unit was correct and the research studies proposed should be commissioned. This epitomised some of the early problems facing HSR. Methods to tackle the evolution of services had already been developed for trials of medical treatments, by undertaking randomised controlled studies in which there was a comparison between those receiving a new drug and those receiving the old drug or method of treatment. This had been accepted by most of the medical profession and Professor Archie Cochrane, in his 1971 Rock Carling lecture, promoted the thesis that this form of controlled trial should also be used in the planning of health services.[6]

There are basic difficulties in evaluating complex services and these include the timing of the evaluation, the number of activities to be covered by the experiment and the nature of the comparison. An important question is whether a theoretical, mathematical or even computer-operated model can be developed to allow the functioning of complex services to be investigated theoretically, before they are put into practice even as trials. Referring to the Rothschild Report[7], the ideal client for a research team would be an individual with a well-defined power to facilitate research and implement the findings who is committed to doing so, because of his or her personal investment in the particular project. The NHS, with its tripartite administrative structure at that time and with widely diffused decision-making, was not such a client. The Department of Health considered itself to be such a client although it had no powers to implement any research! Many individuals within the service welcomed the help of researchers and were often willing to give their time to agree on a plan of work. However, experience with simpler developments showed how difficult it was to obtain this agreement in practice. Although joint planning committees were set up to deal with new developments, it was often difficult if not impossible to get all of them to agree. In the planning of services there is often overlap between authorities with different statutory responsibilities – for example, health (part of the NHS) and social services (part of local authorities) in the long-term care of disabled people.

The early development of research and areas of investigation are described in *Portfolio for Health Volume 1* which gives an excellent description of how the Department of Health attempted to mount a coherent research programme.[8] There were various conditions and situations in which the first such research began, such as screening for disease, research into nursing problems, nutrition, laboratory automation and coronary heart disease.

The field of HSR is vast – it can be classified in terms of methods of investigation used or problems tackled. Catalogues of what was done are included in the annual reports of the Department of Health, in the publications of general journals such as the *British Medical Journal*, *Lancet, Social Science and Medicine* as well as specialist journals such as *Medical Care, Journal of Health Services Research, International Journal of Epidemiology* and *Journal of Epidemiology and Community Health*. It would be difficult and not productive to pick and choose from these. I have, therefore, chosen a different path – that of describing and discussing the problems tackled by one unit, the Social Medicine and Health Services Research Unit at St Thomas' Hospital Medical School with which I am obviously very familiar. In what follows I will describe not only the research carried out, but how it arose and what happened to the findings.

NEED FOR MEDICAL CARE

A fundamental task for HSR is to try to define the need for medical/ health care, assess access and evaluate how the NHS performs in relation to the needs identified. I have already described the differences between need and demand.[9] Most investigations in HSR are concerned with the satisfaction of demands – relatively few address need, in particular unmet need.

St Thomas' Hospital had been severely damaged in the bombing of London during the Second World War. Decisions on rebuilding the damaged hospital were protracted – partly because it was on a prime site opposite the Houses of Parliament on the Thames but also because of the urgent priorities in rebuilding damaged housing which left few material or financial resources for other purposes. There was conflict between politicians. Some wanted the retention of a hospital. Others – for example Herbert Morrison – considered that such a prime site should be used to build a Government Hospitality Centre. Others again, including the then Minister of Health Aneurin Bevan, wanted it to move to where the population was and suggested the site of Wilson's Grammar School in Tooting. The matter was resolved by Sir Allen Daley, County Medical Officer for the London County Council and father of a consultant cardiologist at St Thomas', Dr Raymond Daley. He prevailed on his former boss, Herbert Morrison to press for the hospital to remain where it was.

The decision to rebuild the hospital on the old site was taken at the end of the 1940s but resources to rebuild were not then available. Rebuilding started in 1963, after numerous different plans had been presented. Rebuilding was to occur in several phases. Phase I was completed by the end of the 1960s, but Phase II did not start until 1973–1974 and further phases were abandoned because of the lack of money. The administration and medical staff were concerned to ensure that the rebuilt hospital was capable of meeting the future needs of the NHS and many discussions were held on the buildings required to house a variety of predicted technical machines for diagnosis and treatment. But the fundamental question of what and how much care should/could be provided was the subject of intense debate in which I participated.

As an epidemiologist I considered that the only valid way to determine the need for a service for a specific condition was to identify the number of individuals requiring treatment in a defined population. St Thomas' had always considered that it had responsibility for providing services to its local population in Lambeth. At that time (1963–1967) specialist services were regarded as an adjunct of the general hospital services, most physicians and surgeons saw themselves as generalists with special interests – for example, in cardiology, gastroenterology, urology, colorectal surgery. Since it was impossible to identify all medical needs, I suggested that a number of 'indicator' conditions could serve as a proxy to identify health care needs in a population – cardiorespiratory disease, the most common cause of morbidity and mortality, to reflect the need for inpatient services; peptic ulceration to reflect the need for diagnostic and outpatient services; disability to reflect the need for complex medical and social/community services; and skin disease to reflect the need for skilled, specialist outpatient services. We also chose conditions for which it was possible to measure prevalence with validated methods in the community.

We needed a base population of between 5000 and 10 000 adults to be able to identify a sufficient number of individuals with the various conditions we had chosen to study. Preliminary analysis of a variety of population databases – for example, the electoral roll and the executive council register which provided the basis for registering patients with a general practitioner – were shown to be too inaccurate because of migration and population mobility. It was, therefore, felt necessary to undertake a private census of individuals in a defined group of households and a register of dwelling units in the Borough of Lambeth was available for use as a sampling frame.

This was a major undertaking and although St Thomas' Hospital required the information it did not have the resources to pay for such a large study. The Medical Research Council was approached for funding but felt that such a study required a dedicated research unit. Although a formal grant application might be successful, the Medical Research Council considered that the creation of another research unit in London was extremely unlikely, but that siting and undertaking the work in the provinces might be viewed favourably. Professor J.N. (Jerry) Morris was Professor of Social Medicine and Director of the Medical Research Council Social Medicine Research Unit at the London Hospital and had been involved in the discussions. He advised me to approach the Department of Health who at that time were interested in developing HSR. Their adviser in epidemiology and medical statistics was Sir Austin Bradford Hill in whose department I had worked at the LSHTM. I went to discuss my proposal with him and he was receptive to the idea and urged me to talk to Dr R.H.L. (Dick) Cohen, who was Deputy Chief Medical Officer to Sir George Godber.

At the same time St Thomas' Hospital had a clear interest in supporting the research since it was intended to inform the building and service provision of the new hospital. Equally, the Department of Health was anxious that St Thomas' and its administration were involved and would use the research output. St Thomas' had a wealthy Endowment Fund which did give grants for medical research – these were not large, however, since the funds were mainly allocated toward the rebuilding and the provision of services to the population and hospital staff. The sums of money required to undertake the need studies were large, and well above the normal research disbursement from endowment funds. The Clerk of the Governors of St Thomas', Bryan McSwiney, agreed that I should apply for funding from the Department of Health but that the Hospital's Endowment Fund would underwrite the sum. It thus became possible for us to recruit the necessary staff for the design of the study, the fieldwork and the analysis of the results without waiting for the result of a protracted review. Fortunately, the Department of Health considered that the research was worthwhile and they supported the creation of a research unit at St Thomas'.

The first major study was to be the assessment of medical/health care needs in the local population. The Hospital and the Medical School recognised that a unit concerned with population research was a novelty – most research undertaken in medical institutions, other than the LSHTM, were laboratory or hospital based. Thus the accolade given to our proposed unit and study through an external review process meant that it became respectable and the fact that it was funded externally meant that we were not forced to compete for the limited research endowment funds available.

This means of obtaining resources for HSR served as a model for the future. Almost all the research the St Thomas' Unit carried out was funded by grants that were open to national competition and were reviewed by outside experts.

LAMBETH STUDIES

Local Population Census

A private census, undertaken 1964–1965, was essential as a foundation for all the future studies. We had to identify around 6000 individuals from a population of about 100 000 in the northernmost wards of Lambeth and this would have been a major undertaking for a small Department of Clinical Epidemiology and Social Medicine. The creation in the Department of a Health Services Research Unit was an enormous help. We were able to recruit additional epidemiologists, statisticians and sociologists as well as a number of fieldworkers, mainly nurses, often with health visitor training. Our permanent staff was, obviously, quite unable to undertake the necessary field visits to such a large sample of people so we decided to do this during the Easter vacation and recruited a number of second year medical students, as well as social science students from Bedford College. This was successful in carrying out the necessary fieldwork and also helped to interest both medical and social science students in such research. Several of these students later became academic researchers in the field.

The fieldwork was organised in three waves. First, visits were made by the students, supervised by the permanent staff. Households that failed to cooperate were visited by the permanent fieldwork staff and, if they also met resistance, a third visit was made by me or my deputy director. The census was very successful – more than 98 per cent of the households invited participated.[10, 11] The study was welcomed by the local population who identified themselves with St Thomas' and appreciated our research. We heard some interesting tales of their experiences in the hospital and of members of staff. The very small group of individuals who refused absolutely to participate was a group of market traders who lived locally in a concentrated area in one part of the borough. They admitted openly and in a perfectly friendly way that they did not wish to be recorded in any official document since this might come to the attention of the tax authorities. They said that they trusted us completely – but nonetheless!

Specific Studies

Disability and hospital utilisation
All individuals included in the census completed a brief questionnaire on disability and use of hospitals.[12–14]

Chronic cardiorespiratory disease
The prevalence of chronic cardiorespiratory disease in a random sample of the population was measured by inviting the chosen individuals to visit a clinic which we established for a number of days in the borough. Each individual answered questions on respiratory and cardiac symptoms administered by trained observers. In addition lung function, height, weight, skinfold thickness and blood pressure were measured and an electrocardiogram (ECG) recorded. Details were also obtained of health care received in both hospital and general practice.[15, 16]

Skin disease

This condition had been chosen to reflect the use of outpatient and general practitioner services. A random sample of the population was visited by a medical practitioner trained to identify skin disease and make a diagnosis.[17] Photographs were taken for validation of comparability between the observers and validity of the classification of the lesions which were identified.

Peptic ulceration

This condition had been chosen to reflect the use of both outpatient and inpatient services as well as the adequacy of diagnostic (radiology) services. Unfortunately, it was found that the methods of identification of individuals with a peptic ulcer under the community survey conditions were not as good as expected. The incidence of peptic ulceration had fallen considerably so it was no longer as good a measure of health care needs as we had hoped.[18]

Conclusion on the Lambeth Studies

The feasibility of a series of field studies, including a private census, was demonstrated. The population welcomed the investigation and outstanding cooperation and responses were achieved. Thus accurate figures became available of the prevalence of disability, chronic cardiorespiratory disease and skin disease. The studies were influential in recruiting both medical and social scientists to take an interest in community studies. Information was obtained on the use of hospital services by the local population. The studies demonstrated that current hospital services seemed to be adequate to meet population needs in all ages and social groups. It was clear, however, that the services for the chronically disabled in the local community were not adequate and that the records and services of general practice locally were not appropriate or sufficient to provide the information needed to enable a continuing audit of the adequacy and quality of community care. Those responsible for local hospital and general practice health services, as well as social services, recognised that a greater degree of coordination was needed. Largely as a result of these studies, St Thomas' Hospital created a Committee of Community Medicine linking hospital, general practice and local authority services to take responsibility for identifying gaps in the necessary services and filling them. The Board of Governors, the Medical School and the Special Trustees of St Thomas' recognised the need for development of general practice in Lambeth and supported such developments.

EVALUATION OF SERVICES

In the 1960s, when the rebuilding of hospitals was being considered, the Department of Health decided that new hospitals should be built not only to replace outdated institutions but to enable changes in the pattern of health care to be introduced. It was envisaged that there should be rather fewer inpatient beds and that hospitals should have larger outpatient and laboratory/diagnostic facilities. Patients should, therefore, spend less time in hospital and diagnosis by specialists would occur more often in outpatient facilities with more emphasis on care in the community. Two prototype hospitals were to be built to examine these changes in practice, in Frimley, on the Surrey/Hampshire border and in Bury St Edmunds, Suffolk.

The Research Unit at St Thomas' was invited to put forward proposals for the evaluation of Frimley Hospital. The research proposed by St Thomas' related to a number of discrete problems since we did not believe that a holistic approach was feasible. The Frimley Studies covered four main areas of concern – short-stay after surgery, care of stroke patients, psychiatric care and acute hospital care.

Frimley Studies

Short-stay after surgery

There was some evidence that early discharge after certain surgical procedures would not be harmful and, together with local surgeons, we decided to look at hernia and varicose vein operations. The practice at that time (1969) was that patients would remain in hospital for seven to ten days after operation. We persuaded the local surgeons to undertake a randomised controlled trial in which half the patients were discharged after one to two days, the others after seven to ten days.[3, 19-23]

The main findings of this study were that the change in pattern of care did no harm and the early discharge patients had no more complications than those in the control group. Disappointingly, however, the change in practice did not result in any major savings in either NHS or total social costs. NHS costs were not reduced markedly, partly because the administration did not close the beds that had been used for the post-operative care of early discharge patients but used them for other patients. And since patients discharged early were not available for such tasks as distributing the tea, more nurses and other ward staff were needed. The reason for the small difference in total 'social cost' between the two groups of patients was largely due to the social security costs of time off work for the patient. Both groups had almost the same number of days off work, about six weeks after the operation, irrespective of whether they were discharged early or late. The costs of home care – visiting patients in hospital, time off work for the partner or other relative needed to care for the patient at home immediately after the operation – were small in relation to the cost of social security payments. There seemed to be little rationale for the time taken off work – it was customary to be off for six weeks regardless of the rate of recovery. If the objective was to save money, therefore, it was far more important to consider appropriate time off work than the use of hospital resources. This was not a message welcomed by the Department of Health, and no further research was commissioned to determine the optimal time off work after an operation. Length of hospital stay has shortened. Time off work has also diminished but the latter has probably been partly due to changes in employment with far less manual and more sedentary work as well as to increased direct and indirect pressure on individuals, as a result of the rise in unemployment in the 1980s.

Care of stroke patients
All general practitioners in the proposed Frimley catchment area (a population of 220 000) were invited to notify us of any patient who developed a stroke over a one year period. The study covered all patients who suffered a stroke of sufficient severity to need time off work and medical or nursing care. All patients on the lists of these GPs who died and were found at post-mortem to have died from cerebrovascular disease were included. The type of care received and the place in which this care was provided were recorded, as was the patient's functional ability before and at specified time intervals after the stroke. The objective was to identify met and unmet needs for medical care and to record how these needs were met by hospitals, GPs and local authorities. The study defined the problems of disability that developed after a stroke and provided guides to the services needed for the rehabilitation of patients.[5]

Psychiatric care
A study was carried out on patients in Park Prewitt, a large psychiatric hospital, near Basingstoke, Hampshire in the area of the proposed new Frimley District General Hospital. Changes were occurring both in the development of community psychiatric care and the use of the District General Hospital for acute psychiatry. It was considered that many of the hospital psychiatric patients could function adequately in the community. The selection of patients suitable for life in the community was, however,

difficult since no single individual could be aware of the precise abilities of large numbers of long-stay patients. A questionnaire was, therefore, developed which enabled a study to be made of the functional ability in the approximately 1400 patients in Park Prewitt and this proved useful in identifying individuals who could safely be allowed to live in the community. But the research revealed an unforeseen problem. A considerable number of the long-stay residents in this hospital had been there for a very long time, many for more than 50 years. They had been admitted from a large number of geographical areas, few from the local area. They had lost all contact both with their families, as well as with the community from which they originated. This posed major problems for the provision of community facilities for their care after discharge, as well as the unwillingness of local authorities to take over responsibilities for individuals from outside their own area. The closure of Park Prewitt Hospital was, therefore, a far more complicated and protracted undertaking than had been envisaged, as discussed later in the chapter. This problem was not confined to the Frimley/Basingstoke area but was found also with most other large psychiatric hospitals. They had served a true asylum function and the change to community care was far more difficult than had been expected.[1, 2]

Acute hospital care

Frimley Hospital was in an area that was served by several small local hospitals which were to be closed when the new District General Hospital opened. For many years local GPs had had access to these small hospitals whose consultant medical staff accepted and welcomed this involvement. On the opening of the new hospital the GPs wished to be able to continue to undertake inpatient care with the active agreement of the consultants. The facilities required to provide this GP care in the new hospital needed definition. A study was carried out which described all medical patients from a defined area receiving inpatient hospital care under consultants or GPs, to find out what types of patients were being admitted and what types of care they received in the two groups. It was found that, although GPs and consultants tended to admit the same diagnostic mix of patients, they were using hospital inpatient beds for quite different types of patients. Patients admitted under the care of a GP tended to be older, to be in more terminal stages of illness and to require fewer diagnostic facilities than those admitted under consultant care. Methods were thus devised to define more clearly the precise type of patient for whom such facilities were essential and the approximate size of such facilities.[4, 24]

Conclusion on the Frimley Studies

These studies demonstrated that changing the balance of care from inpatient to community was safe and feasible – even if no great financial savings were made. They provided guidance to planners, administrators and clinicians on how to best change the pattern of care – and some prerequisites. Departmental policies were shown to be sensible but difficulties in their implementation – for example, in the area of psychiatric care – were identified.

ADDITIONAL STUDIES

In addition to these studies of the provision of health services to specific areas, we also undertook studies on individual services.

Screening/Early Diagnosis

Screening – that is, actively identifying a disease or pre-disease condition in individuals who presume themselves to be healthy, but may benefit from early treatment – has always been attractive to both the medical profession and the general population.

The benefits of screening were first demonstrated by the use of mass miniature radiography for the identification of individuals with tuberculosis. With the introduction of effective treatment for this condition after the end of the Second World War, the use of mass miniature radiography became widespread in many Western countries, particularly in the US and the UK in 1947. The background, principles and practice of screening/early diagnosis have been described at length above.[25, 26]

In the early 1960s the Department of Health recognised that the question of screening was likely to be an important development in the delivery of health services. In 1963, Dr J.M.G. (Max) Wilson undertook a prolonged visit to the US to learn of the practice, problems and solutions in a country where screening was already common.[27] Wilson's critical analysis of the possibilities of screening served as a major catalyst for consideration of this method of health service delivery. He and Jungner, a clinical biochemist, published a landmark monograph on the subject for the World Health Organisation.[28]

There had been a number of experiments in the development of screening in the UK. The use of a single visit to a doctor or clinic and the application of multiple tests to the individual was particularly attractive. One novel example was pioneered in 1965 by the Medical Officer of

Health in Rotherham, Yorkshire, Dr Paddy Donaldson. For three summer weeks public health staff opened clinics and invited the population to have a series of investigations – for example, clinical examination, chest X-ray, blood pressure and ECG. These clinics were very popular but they failed in their purpose of improving health in Rotherham for three main reasons. First, the results of the investigations were communicated only to the individuals and not to their GPs so that there was little or no follow-up or treatment. Second, the volunteers who attended the screening clinics were mainly women – few of the male population attended. In the 1960s Rotherham was a town with a great deal of heavy industry, coal and steel so those at most risk failed to receive the service. Third, during the period of the surveys all public health staff were engaged in the screening clinics and no other public health work was done.

Wilson and others recognised these problems. In view of the organisation of the NHS, it seemed that the best way of ensuring that appropriate screening was carried out and that the results of the examinations resulted in treatment where and when necessary was to use the established general practice system. Wilson approached a number of GPs to seek their involvement but was met with a cool reception. The GPs feared that this would entail an increase in their workload and few had organised practices capable of undertaking the task. He, therefore, approached the St Thomas' Unit to see if we could plan and coordinate a proper trial of multiphasic screening in general practice.

The Unit welcomed this approach but soon found that setting up a proper randomised controlled trial in general practice was more difficult than envisaged. None of the practices that had moved to some of the new health centres were interested, in part because the idea of doing a randomised controlled trial in general practice was unusual at that time (1967–1969). Eventually we found a group general practice in St Paul's Cray, Kent, led by Dr John Woodall, which was keen to participate although the number of patients on their list was not sufficient for our purposes. It was, therefore, decided to recruit a neighbouring group practice, which would provide an adequate number of patients for the trial. This practice, however, required payment for the work involved. After discussions with the Department of Health and the two practices, it was agreed that the second practice would receive payment and an acknowledgement while the Woodall practice would be full partners in the research and the principals would be co-authors of any publications.

The randomised controlled trial of multiphasic screening in Kent was successful. All individuals aged 40–64 years in 1967 were identified and then allocated randomly by family and within a general practitioner list into two equal groups, designated 'control' and 'screening'. The screening group, numbering 3297, was invited by personal letter from their GP to be screened. The overall response rate of those attending for screening was 73 per cent. After screening all information was passed to the GP who then carried out a physical examination on each subject and decided on further tests, diagnosis and treatment as appropriate. On average, 2.3 diseases, or conditions, were found per person screened. Fifty-three per cent of this morbidity was not previously known to the GP. Ninety-five per cent of these unknown abnormalities were of a minor nature, being neither disabling nor life-threatening. Of the serious conditions discovered by screening, 56.3 per cent were already known to the GP. Of equal importance to these findings was the observation that for the majority of abnormalities revealed by screening, with the notable exception of anaemia and hypertension, very little new treatment was introduced. All those considered obese were advised to slim and all those who said they were smokers were advised to give it up. The same group of patients were invited to re-attend the screening clinic in 1969. The response this time was somewhat lower, 65.6 per cent, and the yield of conditions was likewise lower than at the initial screening. Both the control and screening groups were examined after seven years and their level of function – blood pressure, lung function, mobility – was assessed. Many different outcome measurements were examined to assess change. Throughout the period of study, data were continuously recorded on general practitioner consultations, periods of certified sickness absence, use of home helps and hospitalisation. Data were also collected on outpatient/clinic attendances as well as use of diagnostic examinations. Deaths (including cause) and departures from the study were recorded. Overall, the mortality in the screening and control group was not significantly different. There were no differences between the two groups in any of the various causes of death. There were no significant differences in certified sickness absence, use of home helps or hospitalisation. There appeared to be a higher overall consultation rate in the screening population but that could have been because of the need to investigate the findings of the screening examinations. The cost of screening was measured and it was shown that, if introduced in the total population, it could increase the costs of the NHS by about 10 per cent, largely because of the examinations which had to be done following the screening. Thus the value of multiphasic screening in this population within the NHS was very dubious.[29–33]

The results of this study were accepted by the Department of Health and no attempt was made to introduce multiphasic screening in general practice. Instead specific nationwide screening programmes have been introduced to identify the early stages, for example, of cancers of the cervix and breast. For raised blood pressure opportunistic screening (case-finding) was advocated. Most adults visit their GP at least once a year and virtually all adults visit their GP once in five years, therefore it was recommended that the visit should be used to measure the patient's blood pressure. The Department of Health also introduced an independent National Screening Committee to review and approve screening procedures within the NHS.[25, 26]

The results of this study have not prevented the private sector, particularly BUPA, from advocating multiphasic screening examinations in middle-age and including this as a benefit in some of their health plans. The concept of this type of screening was popular in the medical profession at the time of this study. Take-up by the population was, however, generally low.

Since about 2000 the medical profession has become far more cautious in promoting this form of screening. Perhaps they have become convinced by the evidence since no trial of such screening has been shown to be effective in improving health.[27] By contrast, the general population in the UK has become more enthusiastic, as shown by the take-up of screening in privately run clinics, often established in supermarket car parks. In the late 1980s the Conservative Government considered introducing multiphasic screening and was only prevented from doing so by concerted resistance from a number of well-respected general practitioners. In 2009, the Labour Government introduced a scheme of preventing cardiovascular disease in individuals in a form of multiphasic screening. The justification for this was based on a number of economic models and field trials of the process, without any practical evidence of effectiveness. It has not been endorsed by the independent National Screening Committee.[27]

The commercial pressures to introduce screening for disease from advertisers and industry including pharmaceutical companies has been detailed.[26] The concept of a 'disease MOT' is very attractive. The success of the South-East London Screening Study in influencing government policy for at least ten years to prevent the introduction of an unproven method is noteworthy. The continuing pressure for the measure by industry and its superficial attractiveness to policy-makers does mean that the evidence gathered in the 1970s in the UK and elsewhere risks being overlooked or considered to be outdated. Those responsible for commissioning and undertaking these studies have retired and no longer have any authority. Few decision-makers have any knowledge of the trials undertaken and the reasons for rejection of the method. That a properly designed randomised controlled trial gives a particular result at one point in time should not preclude further subsequent studies. But it does reinforce the need for adequate valid studies in later years to confirm or refute the results of the original randomised controlled trial.

Laboratory Automation

The trial of multiphasic screening in general practice indicated the need to scrutinise carefully related activities in hospital such as laboratory automation.

Research on screening in the 1960s and 1970s was linked to laboratory automation. This period saw the development of techniques or instruments that could undertake a large number of biochemical tests simultaneously on one sample of blood and thus simplified the process of laboratory examination. A patient admitted to hospital could provide a single sample of blood from which anything from three to 20 determinations could be made.

But this gave rise to a number of important questions. What, for example, was the best organisation and method of working for efficient laboratory services? Could laboratory services be centralised? Did the automation of laboratory tests mean that expert clinical pathologists were no longer required? Could it be left purely to clinicians to interpret the results? What tests should be included in these investigations and what populations would be needed to sustain one such instrument? What automated facilities should be provided for hospitals and what were the staffing, transport and other cost implications? How did these questions affect the design of laboratories?

The development of machines for the automation of biochemical results was fairly simple as was the automation of analysis of blood for haemoglobin, blood cell counts and so on. Automation of bacteriological examinations was far more difficult and automation of histological examination more so. Even now, we do not really have adequate facilities for the investigation of cytological material to a satisfactory standard. A vast array of researchable health service questions thus arose. Would such laboratory automation improve the standards of medical care and outcome and possibly reduce lengths of stay in hospital? There were also questions about the comparability of results and the maintenance of standards of determination.

The Department of Health commissioned a series of studies in various laboratories using automated equipment. Major studies were carried out by Professor Tom Whitehead at the Wolfson Laboratory in Birmingham.[34,35] Other experiments were undertaken at Hammersmith Hospital and various other locations throughout the country. The introduction of such automated procedures in the investigation of patients obviously had or could have serious implications for the care of individual patients. Junior doctors, seeking to impress their senior colleagues, could be tempted to request a complete automated analysis of blood samples for all patients. This might mean anything up to 20 individual tests, many of which would not be relevant in every case and some of which, by chance alone, might return a supposedly abnormal result. This would then require further investigation to confirm or negate the result. It soon became clear that the introduction of automated testing did not lead to reduced lengths of stay or improved patient care. Various studies showed beyond doubt that the use of 20 simultaneous tests without a clear hypothesis for what was actually required in a particular patient was not an economical use of laboratory facilities and that automated equipment could and should be used more efficiently and effectively.

Evaluation of Expensive Technology

In the early 1980s, the possibility of new and expensive technology being introduced into the NHS also required evaluation.

Lithotripsy

One example of this can be seen in the treatment of upper urinary tract stones which changed greatly at this time. First came the development of percutaneous renal surgery and then the introduction of the lithotripter, a machine which can destroy certain types of renal stones without open surgery. Conventional operations to remove upper urinary tract stones were lengthy, costly and associated with appreciable morbidity.

The lithotripter was developed in the Federal Republic of Germany by Dornier Ltd from technology originally designed for offensive warfare. Ultrasonic shockwaves were found to be useless for destroying buildings. They were, however, capable of fragmenting renal stones, first *in vitro* and then in experimental animals. The use of the technique in human subjects was pioneered in Munich and the machine began to be marketed all over the world. When first introduced in Germany, there was no proper evaluation. Urologists in the UK became interested but the machine was extremely expensive – about £250 000 plus running costs. One machine had been bought by a group of urologists working privately in Harley Street, London. One St Thomas' urological surgeon felt strongly that it should be available for use in the NHS and he persuaded the Hospital Endowment Fund to purchase one machine for this purpose.

The Department of Health was approached by St Thomas' Hospital to determine whether they would approve of this purchase and also whether they would contribute to its capital costs. The St Thomas' Health Services Research Unit was brought into the discussion by the surgeon who suggested that a proper randomised controlled trial should be undertaken in order to evaluate and demonstrate how good the machine was. We agreed because the opportunity to do a randomised controlled trial on such an expensive piece of equipment was a golden opportunity to demonstrate how the methodology could be used for the evaluation of techniques in surgery, but also because it was felt that this was an important question.

The surgeon and members of St Thomas' Health Services Research Unit discussed the problem with a large number of urologists in the UK and they all agreed to participate in a trial. As a result, a meeting was held at the Department of Health, chaired by the Chief Scientist, to agree a protocol for the evaluation. It was envisaged that patients needing to have their upper renal stones removed should be allocated, at random, on referral, to either receiving lithotripsy or percutaneous nephrolithotomy, a method developed in the UK at the Middlesex Hospital in London and in Aberdeen.

Various outcome indicators were chosen. It was not considered ethical for patients to be randomly allocated to conventional old-style treatment since this was such an invasive procedure. The agreement between us and the surgeons was that patients in the participating centre would be allocated at random to be treated by lithotripsy at St Thomas' or by percutaneous nephrolithotomy elsewhere. Unfortunately, at the formal meeting at the Department of Health, the surgeons decided, on so-called ethical grounds, that they could not to take part in a randomised controlled trial.

In view of the importance of this machine and its major cost, the Department of Health still urged us to undertake an evaluation using the same method of outcome measurement on patients subjected to litho-tripsy or percutaneous nephrolithotomy. Lithotripsy was to be done at St Thomas', percutaneous nephrolithotomy at other institutions experienced with this methodology. It was considered that since the patients under-going the two procedures would be very similar, an evaluation would still be worthwhile. The criterion of freedom from renal stones, as judged by X-ray, was the major outcome measure used. After a two-year compari-son, the percutaneous technology was shown to be superior to lithotripsy. Economic analysis, sensitive to assumptions made concerning costs, particularly the assumptions about capital costs, since the machines were becoming cheaper, also demonstrated that lithotripsy was not superior to percutaneous nephrolithotomy.

The impact of this research on the diffusion of lithotripsy was limited. The Department was subjected to great pressure from surgeons who wanted to have this new technology in their institution and the purchase of these very expensive machines in the UK and elsewhere continued. In Germany, where the machine had been discovered and developed, more than 30 machines were purchased initially and were described as 'machines in search of stones'. The same occurred in the UK and this led eventually to a proper randomised controlled trial. The Medical Research Council undertook a proper randomised controlled trial of lithotripsy but it was limited to patients with smaller renal stones. This was considered as ethical since previously patients with stones of this size would not have been treated surgically at all!

Thus, this particular investigation is a classic example of how clinicians can influence decisions on the use of high technology contrary to evaluative findings. From the patient's point of view, the new methodology was not invasive but it led to more frequent re-admissions and was not less painful than the percutaneous nephrolithotomy – which, however, required great surgical expertise.[36-9]

DNA probes for service use

DNA probes were beginning to be introduced into the NHS in the 1980s and we undertook an evaluation in three leading genetic centres between 1985 and 1990. The aims were to evaluate the DNA technology in terms of the benefits of the service and its costs, and to provide a framework for estimating the resources required to develop the service throughout the country. DNA probes were considered in our evaluation to be a valuable technology for service use. They are a major component of activity in Departments of Clinical Genetics and DNA testing is concentrated in a few conditions. If they are used, we considered that they should be considered as a regional specialty and their cost actually is relatively low in comparison with other developing medical technologies. They provide a powerful tool for increasing carrier risk precision identification in family members and are a good diagnostic test for assessing the probability of the foetus being affected by a number of genetic disorders.

The technology was assessed for its potential to reduce the number of affected births and decrease the termination of unaffected pregnancies. It was shown that for cystic fibrosis and Duchenne muscular dystrophy, DNA probes markedly decreased the number of affected births and unnecessary terminations. In considering the dissemination of the technology, we found that there was a high demand for the service during an initial period of introduction, followed by a decline, until it reached a steady state. If probes are introduced, it is essential also to have good genetic counselling to explain the technology and its implications to couples. Specialists can sometimes over-value the potential of a new technology and it is crucial that clear guidance is given on how to interpret findings.[40 44]

There are different ways of testing for genetic abnormalities. We undertook a study to evaluate different approaches to carrier screening for cystic fibrosis, one of the most common forms of genetic abnormality. In the past, only the birth of an affected baby identified those at risk. Population carrier screening enables couples at risk to be identified before having the affected child. Screening can be carried out either before conception in primary practice, or during pregnancy in antenatal clinics.

Although there have been calls for the introduction of population screening, the frequency of cystic fibrosis births is only 1 in 2500 so that many individuals need to be tested to identify one at risk foetus. For the alternative strategies, purchasers of health care need to know their overall costs, their population coverage and outcomes, and how strategies compare in terms of their cost-effectiveness. Modern day techniques were used to assess the costs and tangible outcomes of each strategy. These tangible outcomes were the numbers of individuals informed of their carrier status, and the number of carriers, carrier couples and cystic fibrosis foetuses identified. Starting with an overall population of 250 000, the 'target' population was first assessed, followed by the proportion of the population becoming aware of the screening service, followed by the proportion of individuals who agreed to be tested. Service outcomes were then estimated. The results explicitly detailed many of the economic advantages and disadvantages of screening. Antenatal strategies are by far the most cost-effective. The unresolved ethical dilemma is whether it is better to screen people before pregnancy, giving 'at risk' couples time to reflect on reproductive decisions, or during pregnancy, when decisions about terminations have to be rushed. A confidential report on the study was submitted to the Cystic Fibrosis Trust and the research was then submitted for publication. Population screening for cystic fibrosis remains under consideration for universal use in the UK at present.

SMOKING AND RESPIRATORY DISEASE

The major health hazard in the 1960s was smoking cigarettes. Between 50 and 60 per cent of the adult population smoked. Research in the UK and elsewhere had already shown the associations between smoking and cancer of the lung, chronic bronchitis (chronic obstructive pulmonary disease, COPD) and cardiovascular disease. The damage caused by smoking had an important impact on both mortality and morbidity and those concerned with any form of health research had an understandable interest in it.

From its start in 1962, the Unit at St Thomas' was involved in a number of studies on the development of respiratory disease in children in Harrow and Kent. In Harrow we were concerned with respiratory illnesses and ventilatory function in children from birth to age five years (see also Chapter 4). This entailed identifying all births in six electoral wards of Harrow over a two-year period (1963–1965) and visiting the identified families within six weeks of birth. During the visit a questionnaire was administered to the parents about their past history, pre-natal, natal and post-natal experiences, and the newborn baby's inspiratory and expiratory flow rate and inspiratory and expiratory volume were measured. These families were then visited regularly at one-year intervals and the mothers questioned about their baby's illness experience, particularly bronchitis and pneumonia, as well as again measuring the baby's ventilatory function. This was done until the child reached the age of five years with excellent cooperation of the families over this time period. The effect of smoking by the mother during pregnancy on the newborn baby (low birthweight, greater susceptibility to respiratory function impairment) was confirmed. It was shown that the baby's respiratory illness rate was also associated with social class and area of residence. A baby that had an illness in its first year of life was more likely to have more respiratory illness in subsequent years. The children who had a history of respiratory illnesses had a lower level of ventilatory function which was 'dose-related' – that is, the more illnesses, the lower the level of lung function – at age five years.[45–7]

To investigate the progression of respiratory disease in children after age five years we collaborated with the Public Health Department of Kent County Council. We chose four areas of Kent differing in a variety of social, environmental and occupational characteristics – Rochester; Malling rural district; Cranbrook, Tenterden and Romney Marsh rural districts; and Tonbridge. The routine school medical examinations at ages five, 11 and 14 years in these areas were used to gather data on respiratory illness and ventilatory function by the normal staff of the School Medical Service. The doctors were trained in the administration of the questionnaires and measurements of lung function by staff from the Unit at St Thomas'. Kent was chosen for this study because the County Medical Officer considered that his staff would benefit from taking part in research. We were delighted because the Kent areas had a wide range of environmental and social conditions and because this offered us an opportunity to collect a large amount of data at little cost to the Unit. Data collection was supervised by Unit staff to ensure standard-isation and thus comparability of findings.[48-53]

An early observation in the Kent study was that children in both the primary and secondary schools received health education on the hazards of smoking.[48] The County Medical Officer was not impressed by the education administered by the staff of the Central Council of Health Education and asked if we could examine this. As a result of this invitation we randomly allocated the schools in our study into two groups – one to receive this education, the other not. There was no difference in smoking habits between the two groups. Much to our surprise the children who admitted to smoking at ages 11–14 years, even one cigarette per week, had more respiratory symptoms than those who did not admit to smoking. This was dose-related – that is, the more cigarettes a child smoked the more symptoms were reported. In addition it was found that the children who had reported a chest illness one year were less likely to smoke in the subsequent year. These findings aroused interest in what factors influenced the smoking of cigarettes in children and how these could be modified.[49,50] Cigarette smoking was more prevalent in boys than girls, more common in mixed than single-sex schools and more common in comprehensive than grammar schools. Irrespective of these factors, a subjective finding was that the quality and character of the head teacher did seem to have an influence – schools with a pleasant cooperative head had lower smoking rates than those where the head was less amenable.

In view of the effect of smoking on respiratory symptoms in children, the Harrow sample, which comprised a much younger cohort, was re-investigated. It was observed that the babies of parents who smoked cigarettes were more likely to develop respiratory illnesses than those of parents who did not, and the effect was greater where both parents smoked. This was also related to the number of cigarettes smoked and was independent of whether the parents had phlegm.[54-7]

The studies of children from birth to five years and then from five to 14 years demonstrated the importance of a variety of personal, familial and environmental factors on the development and progression of respira-tory disease as well as lung function.[58-61] These studies demonstrated a coherent picture of the development of respiratory illnesses and ventil-atory function. The latter was influenced by respiratory illness, the more illnesses the lower the level of function. The earlier respiratory illness occurred the more respiratory illnesses the children had. The major factors that could be altered or influenced and that were associated with respiratory illness in childhood were smoking by the parent in the first year of life, smoking by the child, level of air pollution to which the child was exposed and deprivation. Each of these factors had an independent association.

These findings gave a clear message as to what preventive strategies could be used to prevent the development of respiratory illness. Preventing an infant from exposure to parents' smoking led to the development of educational programmes for parents during pregnancy. This was actually first developed in Norway following the publication of this research – but was later followed in this country. The control of levels of air pollution was being developed in the UK (further studies of the effectiveness of this were done). There was relatively little knowledge of what led children to take up and continue smoking, and thus how to develop appropriate educational programmes. As a result we were encouraged to develop our research on smoking in children.

The St Thomas' Unit was encouraged to put forward a major programme of research on smoking in schoolchildren. As a result, together with the County Medical Officer of Derbyshire, a research proposal was funded jointly by the Department of Health and the Medical Research Council in 1972–1973. The secondary schools in Derbyshire were divided into two equal groups. The first group was to be investigated by annual questionnaires to all schoolchildren aged 11 to 16 years, about 6000 children. They were asked whether they smoked and, if so, how much, a variety of questions on the smoking habits of friends, parents and siblings as well as a series of questions on other habits and attitudes. The second group of schools was kept free of any intervention in the hope that if suitable methods of smoking prevention were indicated they could be tested in these control schools. Because of the interest in smoking in children and young adolescents the study was continued until the original cohort reached age 21 years. The full findings and methods are described in two books[62,63] and numerous publications.[64–85] The major findings of this longitudinal study were that childrens' attitudes changed first – followed by changes in behaviour. Some children (less than ten per cent) were already smokers when they entered secondary school. The frequency of smoking increased gradually until they reached age 16 years. Between the ages of 16 and 21 years there was a marked contrast between those individuals who continued in school or university, those who went to work, and the unemployed. About 50 per cent of the unemployed smoked in contrast to about 25 per cent of those who continued in education or gained full-time employment. A large number of factors influenced the take-up of smoking in these youngsters – the habits of their peers, their family, their social class, their interest in sport and other activities. The annual questioning was directed to identify possible modifiable factors. A model was developed to assess the likelihood of changing smoking behaviours.[62] Unfortunately this showed that even if it was possible to change some of these, the likelihood of smoking take-up would, at best, only be diminished by about 50 per cent. The main lessons from this very thorough study of the take-up of smoking in children and adolescents were:

1.   To influence children's smoking habits it is essential to start informing them while they are in primary school to prevent them being encouraged to start smoking. It is not sufficient to do this only in secondary school so that by the time they enter the latter their attitudes will be against taking up smoking.

2.   The greatest proportionate change in smoking behaviour occurs after a child has left school. Particularly important in influencing smoking behaviour are continuing in education and employment – social and occupational factors are paramount.

3.   The educational process needs modification – instead of learning facts, much more emphasis needs to be placed on reasoning and risk assessment. Children are quite capable of absorbing scientific and biological principles and extrapolating these to their own experiences. In spite of the findings of this study, educationalists, with whom the findings were discussed, were unwilling to introduce any anti-smoking education into primary schools. They were adamant that in view of the prescriptive nature of the primary and secondary syllabus no change could be made to introduce the children to concepts of risk assessment or to help them to avoid taking up smoking.

Alternative Smoking Materials

By the early 1970s the dangers to health of smoking cigarettes was recognised and accepted by governments. The cigarette manufacturers were obviously concerned and began research on tobacco substitutes which might be acceptable. In the UK products were developed by DuPont and ICI.

The Department of Health established an Independent Committee under the chairmanship of Professor Lord Robert Hunter.[86] This Committee, of which I was a member, was 'to advise on the scientific aspects of matters concerning smoking and health'. Its major task was to review the data manufacturers provided on the tobacco substitute materials and assess their safety. Gallaher and Rothmans submitted a product known as

Cytrel and Imperial Tobacco a product labelled *NSM* (*New Smoking Material*). Both materials satisfied the criteria of safety and toxicity which had been developed and the manufacturers were permitted to market cigarettes containing these products in 1977. Once the cigarettes became available, I chaired a subcommittee which devised a series of studies to determine whether they were less hazardous to health. The 'new' cigarettes were a commercial failure. There were two main reasons for this. First, they were not available for sale in sufficient quantity when they were launched. Second, a highly effective campaign was launched by the Health Education Council, led by Group-Captain Mackie, with the message that smoking the new cigarettes was 'like jumping from the 38th floor rather than the 42nd'. As a result, no epidemiological studies were done and the manufacturers stopped distributing these cigarettes. They began instead to develop and market cigarettes with lower tar and nicotine content, as well as modifying them in other subtle ways – for example, with filters, ventilation holes and so on.[87-9]

The tasks of the committee continued and it was decided that these modified products should be subjected to more than laboratory assessment and that this needed outside scientific experimentation. The cost of the field evaluations was to be met from a fund of several million pounds given by the Tobacco Manufacturers to the Department of Health. The Department devolved administration of this money to the Committee who were responsible both for seeking and assessing appropriate investigations. Total funding of the 37 projects funded by the Committee amounted to about £8 million.[89] One of the largest grants was to the Social Medicine and Health Services Research Unit at St Thomas'.

The Unit undertook a randomised controlled trial of respiratory health in individuals who switched from middle-tar to low-tar products.[90, 91] After a preliminary feasibility study, the main study took place between 1985 and 1988. The hypotheses tested were: first, that smoking low-tar cigarettes would produce fewer respiratory symptoms than smoking middle-tar cigarettes; second, that middle-tar smokers who changed to low-tar, low-nicotine cigarettes would compensate by changing the way they smoked by deeper inhalation or by increasing their 'puff' rate in order to get the desired level of nicotine and tar; and third, that middle-tar, middle-nicotine cigarette smokers who changed to low-tar, middle-nicotine cigarettes would not compensate.

This was a large, complicated study (by far the largest controlled trial that I had ever undertaken) in 21 local authority areas in England. Ethical approval for the study was sought in each area. Approval for the study was initially sought and obtained from the main national anti-smoking group, ASH. At the time of this work electoral rolls were available. A systematic random sample of males in each area was chosen – 265 016 individuals received a postal questionnaire asking about age, gender, respiratory symptoms, medication and smoking habits. Respondents were asked to include an empty cigarette packet of the brand they usually smoked so that we could identify the tar level. We asked about gender to exclude names that can be used by both sexes and ensure that we only included males. About 64 per cent (170 310) of the chosen sample responded. Of these 16 580 were male smokers in the 18–44 year age group and 47 per cent (7736) smoked middle-tar cigarettes. Ninety per cent of these individuals (7029) each received a health warning signed by myself. Ten per cent (707) were not sent a warning. They acted as a control group and were not included in the trial. About 10 per cent of the smokers gave up as a result of this warning. Those who continued to smoke were then invited to participate in the trial. Two thousand six hundred and sixty-six men agreed to participate and 1241 (47 per cent) of these had respiratory symptoms at the start. Six hundred and forty-three men completed the trial – that is, 24 per cent of the original group. The men included in the trial were randomly allocated to one of three types of cigarette – low-tar, middle-nicotine cigarettes; middle-tar, middle-nicotine cigarettes; or low-tar, low-nicotine cigarettes. During the six-month trial participants were visited approximately fortnightly. At each visit cigarettes of the appropriate type were sold to the participant at a cost approximately similar to the cost of cigarettes in a discount store. The cigarettes were supplied in plain, white packets carrying a health warning. At the visits the participants were asked about respiratory symptoms and their peak expiratory flow rate was measured. Compliance with smoking the experimental cigarettes was assessed by questions and a sample of 60 per cent were asked to collect the butts of the cigarettes they had smoked (we had marked these). To assess the inhalation of nicotine the group who collected butts were also asked to provide a urine sample in which cotinine and creatinine levels were measured. Adherence to the experimental design was very good. The results of the large, carefully controlled trial showed little, if any, difference either in the development or loss of respiratory symptoms or levels of lung function. The smokers who were switched to a lower-tar, low-nicotine product compensated, by deeper inhalation and more puffs (as shown by urinary cotinine levels), so that they continued to obtain their usual level of nicotine. The smokers of low-tar cigarettes did reduce the amount of tar which they inhaled – but we were unable to show that this was sufficient to influence their respiratory health, either because the reduction was too small, the measure of respiratory health was not sensitive enough or because the trial did not continue for a long enough time.

The conclusion of this large, complex trial was that the modification of tobacco products does not reduce the harm these do. Thus the only policy must be not to smoke. This message has been largely accepted and most government policies are in agreement on this – modification of product has been abandoned by governments as a possible solution although the manufacturers persist with this policy.

Asthma

Asthma has become a major problem in the UK and the St Thomas' Unit was involved in a number of investigations to try to understand more fully the reasons for the increase in prevalence and incidence, as well as the methods of management of the disease.

Asthma is a disease characterised by intermittent attacks of breathlessness and wheeze associated with narrowing of the airways and is most commonly identified in general practice. Despite intensive research over the years, the nature of asthma and its pathogenesis is obscure. The definition of asthma, however, remains contentious and this issue needs to be clarified. There are two ways in which a diagnosis of the condition can be made. The first is by taking clinical history of the patient's symptoms and experiences and possible previous diagnoses given by other doctors. The second is to use physiological studies of bronchial reactivity to specific challenges from particular antigens or non-specific challenges to other substances such as exercise, histamine, methacholine and prostaglandin F. Unfortunately these two methods of diagnosis do not necessarily classify the same patients as asthmatic. This is not altogether surprising as there is good reason to believe that not all asthmatics are suffering from precisely the same disease. Thus to develop appropriate knowledge for epidemiological and health service studies in similar groups of subjects it is necessary to know: (1) those who have symptoms of 'asthma' but whose bronchial reactivity is normal; (2) those who have no symptoms of 'asthma' but whose bronchial reactivity is abnormal; and (3) those who have both symptoms of 'asthma' and abnormal bronchial reactivity.

A feasible method of objective assessment of asthma in individuals for use in epidemiology and HSR is a questionnaire. This was developed by the St Thomas' Unit but needed adequate testing.

The first study, carried out with the Department of Medicine at Southampton University, took place in two villages near Basingstoke and Blandford. It had two main objectives – the first was to validate the questionnaire, the second to describe the distribution of airway response to histamine in an English community and its relationship with the principal suspected risk factors for asthma and airways disease.

The survey showed that waking at night with shortness of breath was a reasonable marker of bronchial hyper-responsiveness, and that bronchial hyper-responsiveness was related to skin sensitivity to common allergies and to smoking, and that each of these relations was modified by age. Bronchial hyper-responsiveness was also related to urinary sodium excretion, supporting the view that dietary sodium might increase airway responsiveness.

There are general epidemiological reasons – based on data for prevalence and incidence of asthma in different African countries and related to its effect on migration within and between these countries – for believing that a high sodium diet might potentiate bronchial reactivity. The studies in Hampshire showed a relationship between bronchial reactivity and sodium excretion. Because of this evidence, experimental studies were undertaken in conjunction with the Department of Medicine at St Thomas'. The experimental data confirmed the findings of the study in Hampshire that there is a strong relationship between salt intake and bronchial hyper-reactivity in men but not in women.

The distribution of asthma varies greatly and far more than would be expected by chance in different parts of the UK. An opportunity to assess the extent of the variations in prevalence was afforded by the smoking trial referred to above. This required that the sample of approximately 250 000 men should be sampled by questionnaire and the opportunity was taken to ask these men about their current symptoms and medication use, using the International Union against Tuberculosis and Lung Disease (IUATLD) questionnaire. This showed that there were significant variations in prevalence in night-time waking with shortness of breath and that these were related to admission rates for asthma. They were also related to asthma mortality rates. This study led to a European Commission Respiratory Health Survey, a form of 'Concerted Action', coordinated from St Thomas', to document the variations in the prevalence of asthma, the prevalence of exposure to known or suspected risk factors for asthma and variations in the management of the condition. It was hypothesised that the prevalence of asthma varied significantly from one area to another and that this variation was determined by the prevalence of sensitisation to common allergens, as shown by skin tests and both total and specific serum IGE level. A further study was undertaken to determine whether asthma symptoms and airway responsiveness were associated with household allergen levels. The objective here was to determine whether it would be worthwhile to undertake studies on the effectiveness and efficiency of reducing allergen exposure in the home.

Allergen exposure in the home and its relationship to respiratory symptoms was tested in a random sample of adults living in Norwich. The study was divided into two stages – a postal questionnaire and a house visit. The questionnaire on respiratory symptoms was sent to 900 adults aged 20–44 years and was returned by 51 per cent. Dust was collected from the homes and analysed for house dust mite and cat allergen. Although there was a relationship between symptoms of asthma and indoor allergens, methods of containment of indoor allergens were not very successful.

In order to improve the care of asthmatics in general practice, an experiment was undertaken to test the effectiveness of an educational package for asthmatics and to introduce a low salt diet. The educational package was intended to be specific to each patient's asthma. The results of the study showed that those on a low salt diet experienced a consistent fall in bronchial responsiveness of the order of 15 per cent sustained over three months but this could not be consistently maintained

We were also asked to undertake an evaluation of a community-based intervention to improve the management of asthma jointly by the Medical Research Council and the Department of Health. An Asthma Research Centre was started in the Greenwich district in February 1994 with the aim of improving the quality of life for patients with asthma by facilitating the implementation of the British Thoracic Society Guidelines for the management of the condition. The evaluation took the form of a randomised controlled trial in which the unit of randomisation was the general practice. After stratification, according to the number of nursing hours available, the prior training of nurses and social class mix of registered patients in 40 practices were randomly allocated to either the intervention or control groups. The major focus of the intervention was the training of nurses to manage patients with asthma according to the British Thoracic Society Guidelines in the setting of GP-based asthma clinics. The main outcome measure was to be the quality of life for patients with asthma in the community. Other outcomes were symptom frequency, time off work, costs and volumes of asthma treatments prescribed, hospital admission rates and A&E attendance rates for asthma. Process evaluation including the information on current treatment, use of flow meters, proposed action in the event of an exacerbation and reporting, and having discussed asthma with a GP or GP nurse. The main method of data collection was a cross-sectional survey performed at baseline and again two years later.[92–106]

These studies provided information and direction for improving the treatment of asthma in the community and also suggested some means of prevention of the disease. They laid the foundation for a very large series of investigations on asthma worldwide, particularly in Europe and have helped to define the policy towards this serious condition for the Department of Health.

It would seem that hospital admission rates for asthma, for instance, are determined to a major extent by variations in the prevalence of disease. This emphasises the need to understand the environmental causes of asthma if effective measures of prevention and control are to be developed. By far the largest study in this area is the European Community Respiratory Health Survey (ECRHS), a comprehensive review of the variations in prevalence of asthma and atopy in Europe and beyond, including six centres in Canada, four in New Zealand and centres in several other countries outside Europe.

The ECRHS has found huge differences in morbidity distribution across Europe, varying from a three-fold difference in sensitivity to common allergens to a 16-fold variation in people receiving current asthma medication. Genetic variations are unlikely to be responsible for these variations. Diet may have a role to play in variations in asthma prevalence; but diets are hopelessly confounded because foods are eaten in differing combination, making assessment of the effect of isolated dietary inputs difficult.

The ECRHS study showed the complexity of identifying the aetiology of asthma and highlighted the multifactorial nature of the condition and the need for further analyses.

The studies demonstrated that it was essential to define the condition uniformly and confirmed that treatment of symptoms and acute episodes was effective in reducing both mortality and morbidity. The importance of smoking, environmental (including occupational) pollution as well as diet was demonstrated – and has led to much further research and methods of prevention.

MENTAL HEALTH

The problems of mental health services in the UK were evident both in terms of treatment and management. Studies had been published in the late 1950s in various different countries suggesting that patients with mental health problems could be better looked after in the community rather than within an institution, and that admission to an institution might be harmful. Mental health institutions had long been a difficulty for governments. The dangers of institutionalising psychiatric patients had been well described and there had been attempts to identify the essential medical elements of hospital practice and to separate these from the social and residential elements which had become the statutory responsibility of local authorities. These changes were included in the Mental Health Act of 1959 which had profound implications for the organisation of psychiatric services.

It was generally agreed that the number of hospital beds required to treat mental illness in the future would be fewer than in the past. A transition from a system based on mental hospitals to one based on units in general hospitals closely coordinated with social services was considered. The scale could be judged by the fact that over 40 per cent of hospital beds in England and Wales in 1959 were filled by patients for whom psychiatrists were responsible. Mental health problems were also one of the most frequent reasons for consultations in general practice, even though it was realised that there were probably many individuals with mental health problems who did not seek help. As a result, the Department of Health encouraged a series of research investigations.

Investigations in a Large Mental Hospital

The St Thomas' Unit was made responsible for a study to determine whether a large psychiatric institution, Park Prewitt Hospital in Basingstoke, could be closed as discussed earlier in this chapter. The study showed that many of the 1400 patients had been in the hospital since their early teens and had no home to return to. Community care for this group of patients would, therefore, be difficult to organise because only about 20 per cent of the patients had any connections in the local area.[1,2] This problem was gradually resolved since many of these were elderly patients who died. But the community care of mental hospital patients has been a perennial problem in the UK since the passage of the Mental Health Act of 1959. A number of hostels were built and there was a major programme of evaluation of changing the care of mental patients to community care but it has been a long process.[107,108] Part of the difficulty was that the regional hospital boards in the 1970s did not prioritise the changes in practice to build new mental health hostels and the money was diverted to acute care.

The Department of Health also encouraged research by Shepherd and his colleagues to undertake a variety of different studies to help general practitioners identify mental health problems in their patients, to use social workers in the care of mental illness and to create registers for the continuing surveillance of patients with mental illnesses.[109]

Shepherd drew attention to the fact that, although about one-seventh of all consultations in general practice are related or attributable to mental health problems, these are often neglected.[110] In his work he emphasised the importance of general practice and illustrated this with the work of Watts in depression who demonstrated that 'the proportion of depressed patients who come to the attention of a psychiatrist is no more than 2.92/1000 of the general population and no more than 1.8 per cent of all depressed people'.[111] Shepherd went on to develop a variety of tools which could be used in mental health care in the community, emphasising the central role of the general practitioner.

The Department of Health recognised the importance of mental health and supported many investigations. Of particular note were studies evaluating community psychiatric services. These were based on a register of individuals in Camberwell by Wing and his colleagues which continued for many years.[112, 113]

Mental illness in the elderly has been a perennial problem and early investigations were undertaken in North London by Mezey and colleagues. An example of an examination of inappropriate organisation and what could be achieved is illustrated by his study in 1968.[114]

Shepherd undertook a variety of studies of psychiatric morbidity in the community from 1965–1980 and also demonstrated the high prevalence of psychiatric disorder among the elderly. These problems were often unrecognised by the patient's GP and, although frequently associated with serious social impairment, were rarely referred to mental health services. His studies were designed to determine the characteristics of psychiatric disorders in the elderly, the severity of the disabilities and the methods of coping and caring for these patients.[109, 115]

One of the largest continuing studies in the field of mental health from the mid-1960s was the series of studies by Dr Albert Kushlick on the provision of services for the mentally handicapped carried out in the Wessex Region (Dorset, Hampshire, Isle of Wight and Wiltshire). The prevalence and severity of mental handicap was measured by epidemiological studies. The findings were then used to provide appropriate services, both domiciliary and residential. The adequacy and effectiveness of the service provision was then evaluated and appropriate changes made if necessary. These investigations were a model of how service provision for a defined population could be provided and have been widely applied in the UK.[116]

A further example of HSR as applied to mental health was the establishment of an Addiction Research Unit under Professor Griffiths Edwards at the Maudsley Hospital, London.[117] Initially the Unit concentrated on the problems of alcohol addiction but it soon developed interests in drug addiction and smoking.

Whereas early HSR and mental health studies were largely descriptive, more recent research from the mid-1980s has involved more emphasis on evaluating and experimenting with varying methods for the provision of mental health services as described by Goldberg and his colleagues.[118]

GENERAL PRACTICE

Since 90 per cent of all patient–doctor contacts occur in general practice, it was obviously important to develop this as a research field. Eimerl commissioned various studies to help develop the work of general practitioners, such as in the use of ancillary staff and in the development of premises.[119] In the early 1970s Eimerl developed a method by which contacts in general practice could be easily recorded and classified – the EBook system. The creation of the Royal College of General Practitioners (RCGP) greatly improved the status of general practice in the 1960s and it became a reputable branch of medicine, with great interest in trying to see how it could be improved. Fry (1922–1994) describes a series of investigations in his practice in South-East London, and showed the way in which research could be applied to the solution of a number of simple problems.[120]

The St Thomas' Research Unit became interested in the development of general practice. The Medical School had as a member of its Council Stephen Taylor, a politician, later to become a Junior Minister in the Labour Government of 1945–1950. He first made his name by being commissioned to undertake studies of general practice by the Nuffield Provincial Hospitals Trust. A number of studies had been undertaken in the UK, which showed the poor quality of general practice in England particularly, and in the UK in general. Taylor was commissioned to probe this further, and he demonstrated some examples of outstanding general practice in a variety of places including in London.

Taylor was a graduate of St Thomas' Hospital Medical School and a great friend of the then Dean, Mr Bob Nevin. Being a member of the Council, he persuaded St Thomas' that it needed to develop general practice as a subject. When I was appointed in 1962 as Senior Lecturer in Clinical Epidemiology and Social Medicine, I was made responsible for teaching general practice. I enlisted the help of John Fry to lecture to medical students about general practice.[120] Fry was not a lecturer who could evoke enthusiasm in his audience. His tone of delivery was somewhat flat and he only came in once a week to deliver his lectures. We, therefore, decided to recruit a full-time teacher in general practice. Taylor and Nevin had already negotiated with Lambeth Council that if a particular part of Lambeth near the Hospital was to be rebuilt, it would include a general practice teaching unit, and location and suitable tenancy and rental arrangements had already been agreed. The main question was who would actually staff this general practice? Taylor had identified a single-handed GP working in Lambeth, Dr George Gage, who was considered to be quite outstanding. It was envisaged that this would be the core general practice teaching unit but academic involvement was also essential. There were no funds available for this so Nevin and I went to see Sir George Godber, the Chief Medical Officer, to ask for his help. He suggested that the Department of Health should add a specific sum to the research budget of the St Thomas' Research Unit to fund an academic senior lecturer in general practice with the initial research remit of evaluating the move to new premises. We were fortunate in attracting Dr David Morrell, a senior lecturer in Edinburgh, to the post. We started a general practice teaching unit in Lambeth Towers, consisting of two practices – Gage and Morrell and Marson and McPherson. We thus had a four GP unit with about 10 000 patients, sufficient to provide the nucleus for both research and teaching. This was the first academic unit in general practice in England. A little later, a similar unit was developed at Guy's Hospital Medical School. All of this was, of course, a forerunner to the major developments in general practice that have taken place since then, with academic units in Manchester, Sheffield and many other places.

Development of HSR in General Practice

Research in general practice has a long history and many clinical advances and knowledge of specific diseases are based on work done in general practice in the UK. Examples of this include James Mackenzie's work on cardiology[121-3] and William Pickles' studies of infectious diseases.[124-6] The first Professor of General Practice, Richard Scott, was appointed by the University of Edinburgh in 1963 but there was little, if any, research in general practice concerned with HSR. One of Richard Scott's Senior Lecturers was David Morrell who was appointed Senior Lecturer in the St Thomas' Social Medicine and Health Services Research Unit in 1967 and Professor in 1973.

The first series of studies, 1968–1970, were of the content of general practice, to demonstrate the differences between medicine in hospital and in the community, and were carried out in the St Thomas' Lambeth Road practice. A detailed study was made of the medical care delivered to a defined population of about 4500 individuals registered with a general practice, over one year. At that time 75 per cent of the population received primary care services annually, 11 per cent were referred to hospital outpatient departments and 1.4 per cent were admitted to hospital as emergencies. This study made it possible to identify the knowledge and skills demanded of a general practitioner and thus to clarify the desirable content for the vocational training for general practice being developed at that time.[127–30]

These studies led to discussions and experiments on the optimum place for delivering different forms of care – antenatal care,[131] diabetes and asthma. The forms of care for these conditions were evaluated by comparisons of patient satisfaction, adherence to appointments, breast-feeding, control of diabetes and so on. With appropriate training, transfer of hospital care to general practice for these conditions was found to be satisfactory; this was tried in two other local practices and was then copied by many others in all parts of the UK.

Transfer of a group practice into new, purpose-built premises also enabled a study to be done on the effect of an appointment system.[132] In 1968 appointment systems in general practice had only just been introduced and there was little information on how they would affect utilisation and health. The study showed that the appointment system led to greater emphasis on delivering medical care to the elderly.

These studies inevitably led to an investigation of medical records in general practice that at that time were A6 forms in envelopes. The records were converted over a period of three months to A4 problem-oriented records and an age–sex and morbidity record was constructed and transferred to a computer. These developments were published and distributed by the RCGP in the form of an Occasional Paper and were widely adopted. At the same time, the advantages of a structured medical record were tested. A group of patients with diabetes and a group with congestive heart failure were identified in the academic practice and a neighbouring control practice. The criteria for good quality care for these patients were established by an independent group of general prac-titioners. A structured record designed to encourage doctors to adhere to the agreed care was developed and introduced into the medical records of the relevant patients attending the academic practice. The process and outcome of care was compared between the patients in this and the control practice over one year. Recording of the process of care was significantly improved in the academic practice. However no significant difference was identified in functional performance, level of disability or other outcomes. As a result of this, a study recommending auditing the care of patients suffering from chronic disease was published by the RCGP – and introduced an element of realism into medical audit.[133, 134]

Demands for medical care for simple conditions such as the common cold do not reflect their incidence. In view of the variation in demands made on general practice by individuals with similar symptoms a study was devised to determine whether demand for care was related to objective measures of anxiety or other social factors. This was done by asking a random sample of women aged 20–45 years to keep diaries of the symptoms they experienced over four weeks. Their demands for care were measured over a period of one year. The statements also described, in a questionnaire, their social setting and their satisfaction with this. The study identified factors influencing demands for medical care and highlighted the importance of self-care in response to each symptom of illness. It led to changes in the attitudes of the British Medical Association, and highlighted the importance of the pharmacist in over-the-counter prescribing for self-care. It also led to initiatives in the education of the general public in the management of common symptoms of illness.[135–137]

In the studies of symptoms in general practice, six symptoms were identified as accounting for 50 per cent of new requests for medical care for children under the age of five years. A booklet was produced designed to allay parental anxiety, to describe the management of these six common symptoms, and to indicate when professional advice should be sought.

The booklet was given, at random, to one-half of the families in the practice with at least one child under age of five years. The other such families did not receive the booklet and formed the control group. The demands for care of the families in the study and control groups were measured. In addition, a sample of patients in the test and control groups was interviewed and their knowledge of the management of the symptoms described was tested. The study group requested significantly fewer home visits than the controls for three of the six symptoms and made fewer requests for medical care for two of the other symptoms. The booklet was printed by the Health Education Council and the demand for it was such that over one million copies were distributed.[138]

One of the most common symptoms patients present to the GP is back pain and in 1979 a Department of Health Working Group identified this as an area requiring investigation. As a result a study was done which included all patients in the practice who presented with low back pain over one year. Two hundred and thirty-seven patients presented over one year with 252 episodes. This study was on the natural history of the symptom, the identification of the clinical features on first presentation which help to predict outcome, and methods of measurement of the outcome. Although there was a general tendency for back pain to improve with time, one-quarter of patients reported increasing disability during the first week and a further one-quarter reported increasing disability during the next three weeks. By the end of four weeks from the initial consultation, almost all patients had stopped consulting and were back at work. But, at this time, only one-third of patients were pain-free and less than one-quarter reported no disability from backache. The most useful predictors of poor outcome, initially, were history of pain lasting for more than a week, pain of gradual onset, restricted straight leg raising and back pain on foot dorsiflexion at the extreme of straight leg raising. A disability questionnaire was a simple, reliable measure of the severity of back pain. Ability to return to work was poorly related to pain and disability. The patients who had had one episode of back pain were three times more likely to consult again for back pain in the subsequent years than the general population.[139, 140]

One result of these studies was the development of a booklet intended to help patients presenting to general practice with back pain. It was helpful to patients and effective in reducing the number of consultations and use of physiotherapy services as well as the number of laminectomies, compared to the control group.

These studies in general practice encouraged the Unit to explore further the ways in which patients could be involved in their own care, particularly for the management of chronic conditions, and to actively involve them in the decisions on their care. For this to succeed, patients require factual information about the nature of the disease, its natural history and the impact of treatment, and also to understand and agree with the doctor on the objectives of their care.

To test this, hypertension was chosen as a common condition whose natural history is reasonably well understood. A booklet was produced for use by patients with this condition and evaluated in a randomised controlled trial in six general practices in South London.[141] The booklet was successful and so a number of other booklets to enable patients to hold their own medical records were devised for the management of other chronic conditions, such as diabetes and asthma.

This research in general practice was dependent on meticulous record keeping. Developments in computer technology in the early 1980s encouraged the introduction and evaluation of the use of computers in the general practice. Studies were carried out: on the introduction of a computer-assisted repeat prescribing programme; on the development of a drug coding scheme designed for the computerisation and audit of prescribing data; on audit in general practice; on the use of district nursing time; on cervical cytology; on immunisation in children aged five years and under; and on recording of major life events.

Psychological and mental health issues are other important causes of consulting a general practitioner and a study was undertaken in 1987–1989 to investigate maternal depression and its effect on childhood development. Two hundred and fifty women from two general practices were recruited in early pregnancy and completed a series of interviews and questionnaires until the end of the first post-natal year. About 20 per cent of the women were found to be affected, mainly with symptoms of depression. More of these episodes were associated with financial problems, bad housing, marital relationships and lack of social support and adverse life events, rather than with medical issues.[142]

A more service-oriented group of studies carried out in 1992–1993 was concerned with the identification of problems associated with the admission of acutely ill patients to London hospitals. Admission to hospital is only possible if beds are freed by discharging patients from the hospital so the study of admissions was complemented with an investigation of discharges from hospital and their impact on community nursing services.

These studies and their results can be summarised as follows:

1. A major problem for hospitals was the unpredictability of demand for acute admission. The greater the pool of beds available, the less likely was it that serious problems would arise. Efficient management was closely related to the status and power of the bed managers and their relationships with the clinicians and nurses. The establishment of 'buffer' beds in an Accident and Emergency Department appeared to facilitate efficient management.[143] These so-called buffer beds were temporary beds in Accident and Emergency used to accommodate patients needing admission and used until a permanent bed became available in a ward.

2. In a study of 493 consecutive acute admissions to hospital by 11 general practitioners in the Lambeth, Lewisham and Southwark Family Health Service Administration (FHSA) over a period of seven weeks, more than one-third of patients (37 per cent) were over 75 years old. The negotiations between the GPs and admitting doctors were very laborious and often confrontational and in more than half (58 per cent) they took over 10 minutes. Problems were encountered in 30 per cent of arrangements for ambulances by 999 calls.[144]

3. A study of adult attendees and admissions was undertaken over a two-week period in the Accident and Emergency Departments of two inner London hospitals and one outside London. The departments were monitored by teams of fieldworkers working on 24 hour rotas. During the study, 3804 attendees and 884 emergency admissions were questioned and observed. Waiting times in all the hospitals were longer than those recommended by the Patient's Charter. All departments were understaffed, particularly in respect of senior staff. Most patients were seen by a Senior House Officer

in training and 40 per cent of these had an X-ray requested. Serious delays in obtaining a second opinion on specialist advice were common and this resulted in delayed admissions. Only 13 per cent of patients in the inner London hospitals were tourists or commuters, compared to 6 per cent outside London. Only 19 per cent of the attendees had not consulted a GP; and of the GP referrals, 75 per cent were accompanied by a letter and 15 per cent had been arranged by telephone. Ten per cent of all admissions were considered to be the result of social factors.[145]

4.   A qualitative study of patients was undertaken on admission to two London hospitals as emergencies. Interviews were carried out on 83 patients following admission. The major findings were the unhappiness of patients about the lack of information on what was happening to them, what was wrong with them and what would be done. They also commented on long periods of time spent on stretchers, inadequate privacy, long periods waiting for pain relief and other disruptive patients. Long waits for ambulances were also reported, although when these arrived the care was good.[146]

5.   In a study of the problems encountered by district nurses as a result of poorly planned discharges in the catchment area of three London Hospitals, semi-structured interviews were conducted with 44 district nurses and data collected on 139 referrals. There were problems with 72 per cent of these referrals: in 23 per cent the district nurse was not informed of the discharge; in 22 per cent discharge was considered inappropriate in view of the patient's social circumstances and condition; 26 per cent of all discharges occurred at weekends; and in 70 per cent of cases less than 48 hours notice of discharge was given.[147]

These last five studies illustrate some of the problems surrounding acute admissions. Their results were widely disseminated by the King's Fund and Department of Health and it is disappointing that these problems are still common today, in spite of a great deal of publicity.

Some Examples of other General Practice Research in the Period 1960 to 1990 [i]

It was at this time that research in general practice began to take off. The first English Chair of General Practice was endowed in Manchester in 1969 and held by Professor Patrick Byrne (1913–1980).[148] This and some

---

[i]   Only illustrative references are quoted.

of the other academic departments – for example, Leicester with Professor Marshal Marinker,[149] and Dundee with Professor Jimmy (D.E.) Knox (1927–2010)[150] – concentrated on developing research on education and communication in general practice. In the early 1970s, the RCGP's General Practice Research Unit in Birmingham under Dr D.L. Crombie,[151] Dr R.J.F.H. Pinsent[152] and Dr D.M. Fleming began to develop a system of recording diseases in a group of general practices which has been of great value in the surveillance of communicable disease. It continues under the direction of Dr Fleming. Dr R.E. Hope Simpson (1908–2003) in Cirencester developed a series of ground-breaking studies of infectious disease in general practice in the early 1970s, making significant advances in our knowledge of the spread of such conditions as herpes zoster, varicella and influenza.[153] The Medical Research Council even funded a virus laboratory in his practice. Dr Ian Gregg (1925–2009) and colleagues in his Roehampton practice developed important studies on the natural history of asthma in the mid-1980s,[154] and Dr C.R. Kay, from general practice in Manchester, coordinated a large study of the risks of oral contraceptives in the early 1980s.[155] The use of general practice for the study of common diseases was recognised by the Medical Research Council who recruited a number of practices to cooperate in studies of the treatment of high blood pressure in the early 1980s.[156] These are just a few examples of general practice research undertaken in the period between 1960 and 1990 but they illustrate that the majority were concerned with clinical rather than HSR and with education and communication.

NUTRITION

The Department of Health has long been responsible for providing scientific advice on national food policy. Many lessons were learnt from experience in the First World War when the UK was considered to be only three weeks away from having an inadequate food supply because of problems with the import of food stuffs and attacks by U-Boats. Between the two world wars, various investigations were undertaken on what constituted an adequate food supply and examples of this research are described in the book by Holland and Stewart on public health.[157] As a result, when the Second World War began the country was prepared and had developed a coherent policy for the rationing of food and providing a balanced diet to the population. In fact, as I have stated on previous occasions, it is possible to argue that food rationing in the Second World

War was responsible for a major improvement in the health status of the British population. After the end of the war, there was still a need to identify problems in nutrition at least in the most vulnerable groups such as children, pregnant women and the elderly, and to devise an appropriate nutritional strategy to protect them. Surveys on nutrition were undertaken jointly by officers of the Department and nutritionists, under the guidance of the Committee on Medical Aspects of Food Policy (COMA). Nutrition surveys were helped greatly by the advent of computers and by the development of technical work such as the production of food tables and codes which were up-to-date and capable of providing information for the analysis of nutritional intake. These tables, based on information from many sources, were prepared in collaboration with colleagues from other departments of state and itemised over 800 food substances. The first time that this was applied was in 1963, with a pilot survey of pre-school children to determine the effectiveness of welfare by looking in this group. The St Thomas' Health Services Research Unit became involved in these studies.

As I have described above, the Unit had undertaken a study of respiratory disease in school children in Kent. One of the measures used was to measure height and weight of the children in the respiratory disease study. This demonstrated that there were wide variations in height and weight of primary school children, and that this was associated with social class.[158] In view of the concern with the nutritional status of children and the need to determine whether school meals and milk were still required by this group, we were encouraged to develop research on the food intake of children. Studies were based on the height, weight and social class which had been recorded in the respiratory disease studies, and about 800 children were recruited to a study in 1968–1969, chosen on the basis of their demographic status – namely age, family size and social class. Each child was given a weighing scale and was asked to record and weigh everything that he or she ate for a week. This was undertaken under the supervision of a qualified nutritionist. The study showed that there was no longer any evidence of malnutrition in children between the ages of five and 14 years in Kent.[159] It did show that children from the lower social class groups, particularly girls, were tending to be obese. The detailed food intake study confirmed the findings of the measurement study – namely that no child was undernourished and that the food intake of the sample of children included in these investigations was adequate. There was some difference between the food intake of different social class groups. In general, the protein intake was greater among the more affluent than among the poorer groups. Since the study had been designed to identify the most vulnerable, there was a relatively large sample of 80 children from single-mother households. Surprisingly, the food intake of the children from single-mother households was better than the equivalent from families in the same social class group, in the same age, with two parents. Thus, this study in the late 1960s demonstrated that there was no evidence in any social class group of undernutrition. If anything, those in the poorer families were as well or better fed than the others, but the problem of obesity was already becoming evident.

With the change in government in 1970, the Conservative Government were concerned with changes in welfare food provision. Mrs Thatcher had been made Secretary of State for Education and she was interested in rebuilding many of the old schools, particularly those used for primary schools. For this, she considered, in view of the lack of evidence for undernutrition, that the welfare food policy for children and pregnant mothers could be changed. This resulted in the withdrawal of free school meals and milk. Many individuals were wedded to the provision of free school milk particularly for pre-school and primary school children and there was a great deal of resistance to this policy. The policy was introduced by the Conservative Government of the day, however, with the proviso that a system of surveillance and research should be established to ensure that the changes in welfare food policy did no harm. Separate investigations were established to examine the effect of the withdrawal of welfare foods in pregnant women, in pre-school children and in primary school children. The primary school children were investigated by the St Thomas' Unit and we established a system of surveillance of nutritional policy in 26 areas in England and Scotland.

Nutritional Surveillance Study

For the Nutritional Surveillance Study (1972–1992), 26 areas in England and Scotland were chosen on the basis of an index of deprivation which was heavily weighted to those areas that were most deprived. The areas were widely scattered throughout the two countries and many of them were in rural areas since poverty was more common in rural than urban areas at that time. To have sufficient numbers to study, we needed about 200–800 school children from each area, so the number of schools involved in an area varied from one to four primary schools, depending on the number of children in a given school. The school children were measured for height and weight every year during their time in school. The study demonstrated that the withdrawal of free school milk had no effect on the health of school children measured by rate of growth. Other measures of health, such as respiratory disease, were also introduced into this study subsequently.[160, 161] The LSHTM undertook studies on pre-school children from birth and again, no ill effects were demonstrated as a result of the withdrawal of free milk. A randomised trial of free milk being provided to primary school children was also undertaken in Wales.[162]

The St Thomas' study was continued annually until 1994 and was considered to be a reasonably successful method of surveillance of the health and growth of primary school children. It was continued to make certain that the changes in the socio-economic circumstances of children, in particular, with withdrawal of free school milk and meals did not do any harm.

The study was used by the Cabinet in order to decide health policy. With the advent of the Labour administration in 1975, their manifesto included the return of free school milk which was a highly emotive subject within the Labour party. Professor Brian Abel Smith, who was the Chairman of the Advisory Committee to the St Thomas' Research Unit, was also an adviser to the Secretary of State for Health when the decision on whether free school milk needed to be reintroduced was being discussed in the Cabinet. Abel Smith approached me to determine whether I felt reintroduction was necessary. I urged him strongly to oppose this since the problem was not under-nutrition but overnutrition. At his behest, I wrote a one page brief to the Secretary of State for Health, David Ennals, to advise him to resist the manifesto commitment on the reintroduction of free school milk. The Secretary of State for Health won the argument and free school milk was not reintroduced. This is the only occasion that I know where research that had been carried out by a research unit directly influenced a Cabinet decision.

By the early 1980s, poverty and deprivation had changed in England and Scotland. It was now greater in urban than rural areas, and the groups considered to be at particular risk were those from ethnic minorities, particularly the immigrant groups from the Indian subcontinent. Because of this, we doubled the number of areas included in the study to 52. This additional sample of 26 areas was weighted towards inner city areas with a large proportion of immigrants. The system of surveillance did not show any changes in levels of nutrition or in health, as measured by changes in height, weight gain or slowing of growth rates. In the last years of the study – that is, in the early 1990s – the only group possibly at risk were girls from the Indian subcontinent, particularly from Gujerat. The sample of children from Gujerat was large enough to identify any effect on this subgroup and a slowing growth with age was shown. A possible explanation for this problem was that children from this group were from very poor households, and for cultural reasons, girls were less valued than boys. Thus the slowing in height and weight gain in girls from Gujerat could be explained that for cultural or other reasons they received less food. This finding was not present in any of the other groups in the study. In all other groups the real health problem was obesity. This was particularly important among girls from low social class groups.

There was a memorable occasion when I gave a public talk on the system of surveillance and the problem of obesity in school children in the Festival Hall, London. The Secretary of State was appalled by my statement and issued a press release to say that there was no problem and I was misguided. Six weeks later the Chief Medical Officer's report referred to the problem of overweight primary school children and emphasised that this was becoming a public health problem! It is salutary to note that the problem of obesity and being overweight was first recorded by us in the late 1960s and continued to be highlighted in our system of surveillance over the years although little notice was taken of these findings for a variety of political and commercial reasons. Our study demonstrating the issue of obesity should have led to intervention in the 1970s and 1980s before it became the serious problem it is today.

DISABILITY

The studies of health care needs of the population of Lambeth had identified the area of disability and the physically disabled as one where there was a deficiency in services provided by the local authority and by the health services. As a result, the Department of Health approached St Thomas' Unit in 1980 to undertake a series of studies on the health and care of the physically disabled in Lambeth which would help to map out the areas where there were problems, and reveal possibilities and opportunities for improving care. The studies had three main aims:

1. To identify a sample of disabled people in Lambeth and to estimate the prevalence of disability.
2. To describe the course of disability over time.
3. To provide information for the strategic planning of health and social services.

The project included: a postal screening study for physical disability; a longitudinal intervention study; a qualitative in-depth study of the social and economic consequences of disability for a small group with rheumatoid arthritis; a value scaling study to measure the perceived severity of the functional limitations and activity restrictions which comprise disability; and a 'priority' study to examine the preference for cash benefits of local authority services held by disabled people, the relatives and friends who care for them, and the planners and providers of services.

Postal Screening Study

The questionnaire used to identify disabled people in Lambeth was piloted in a general practice in Kingston upon Thames. Questionnaires were sent to a sample of patients in a general practice, and between three and six months later, fieldworkers asked to sample disabled and non-disabled respondents using the same questions as those contained in the postal questionnaires. Between eight and 12 months after interview, general practice records were examined and general practitioners completed a screening questionnaire for the respondents under their care. Individuals were classified as disabled if they had difficulty with particular activities of daily living, or a specified medical problem generally associated with disability or had made use of selected formal services in the preceding 12 months.

A comparison of the postal interview and administered questionnaires showed that although a high proportion changed their response to at least one item when being interviewed, there were no changes in disability classification. It was, therefore, concluded that the postal questionnaire formed a reliable screening instrument.[163] General practitioners were shown to know more than they recorded but were aware of only 30 per cent of the disability items reported by their patients. This indicated that their records and knowledge were inadequate for validating disability screening questionnaires and identified that there needed to be greater coordination between the health and social services.

The postal questionnaire was used to identify disabled people aged 16 years and over in Lambeth, with the aim both of providing a sample for further study, in the longitudinal interview study discussed below, and of calculating prevalence. In a previous study in early 1978, a postal questionnaire was sent to a 10 per cent sample of private households and completed by 18 700 people (79 per cent of those eligible). Disability was assessed using 25 screening items which related to ambulatory mobility, body care and movement, sensory motor limitations and social activity.[164]

Prevalence of disability identified in this previous survey was double that of the estimate provided by the 1969 National Survey of Disability.[165] It was found that about 10 per cent of men and 15 per cent of women were classified as disabled in this survey. However, when only 11 screening items, which were broadly comparable to the National Survey, were considered, the estimated prevalence of disability was very similar to the National Survey figure. Items which significantly increased reported disability were sensory motor items, such as frequent falls, and items related to occupation such as difficulty in doing a job of choice or housework. An issue highlighted in these findings, and examined in more detail using the longitudinal disability interview survey, is whether the identification criteria used by local authorities should be broadened to include additional items which significantly increased reported disability. Comparison of responses to specific items with the earlier Lambeth health survey conducted by the St Thomas' Unit also drew attention to the effect of question wording on reported disability. The questions termed in terms of performance or non-performance – that is 'do you do?' – rather than capacity – that is 'are you able to do?'– increased reported disability significantly.

Longitudinal Interview Survey

Longitudinal design is essential for examining the factors influencing the cause of disability. The mentally handicapped, over 75-year-olds and the blind and/or deaf were excluded from the original sample of 1100 disabled and 500 non-disabled people selected from the postal screening study to be followed up. Eighty-one per cent of disabled and 70 per cent of non-disabled people were interviewed in each of the three phases of study over a period of three years from 1978–1981. The questionnaire was used and each wave of interviews contained a core series of questions, plus additional questions on specific areas. A further question-naire was then developed for undertaking the longitudinal study which measured a variety of physical, psychosocial, eating, communication and work limitations. This was tested for its statistical properties and shown to have lower standard errors and greater repeatability than the previous questionnaire and would, therefore, be useful as a summary measure in comparing changes over time in groups of people.[166]

Comparison of the results from this longitudinal questionnaire survey and the findings of surveys from the 1969 National Survey of Disability showed that a number of individuals would not be assessed for need of local authority services for the disabled, carried out under the Section 1 of the Chronically Disabled Person Act of 1970, unless they were housebound or over 69 years of age. Thus, local authorities who use the National Survey measure may not identify many disabled people who experience appreciable to severe restriction in ambulation, mobility and household management, and might be in need of services.[167]

Community-based studies have concentrated on the effects of social ties on the onset of illness, particularly among people who have recently experienced a life crisis. It was thus necessary to look at the influence of social ties on the cause of disability. The relationship between level of social contact and changes in disability among people aged 45 to 75 years was examined, controlling for age, sex and initial level of disability. This indicated that over a two-year period, a low level of social contact was significantly associated with deterioration in psychosocial disability, both in the presence and absence of life events. A similar but weaker pattern existed for physical disability. Such analyses can say little about the process by which social ties exert a protective effect, but nevertheless contributed to the growing body of evidence on the importance of such ties.[168]

In contrast to the view that disabled people, and particularly those living in inner city areas, lack local social ties, the majority of respondents appeared to have developed such ties, with friends and neighbours forming major sources of support. The foreign-born population was, however, distinctive in that they often lived in close proximity to related people, reflecting the general pattern of settlement of recent immigrant groups. The main effect of increasing disability appeared to be in reducing total social contacts rather than influencing the strength of people's main supporting relationships. The lower level of social contact of more severely disabled people largely reflected their restricted activities outside the household, particularly since they had a low rate of labour force participation. Although groups with relatively low levels of support could be identified, what was more striking was the considerable range in support scores. Individuals with a high level of one form of support, such as social contact, were not always associated with the availability of other forms of informal support, such as confiding and helping. This suggests that identifying those people with low levels of informal support is more complex than has generally been recognised. The different forms of support also emphasise the importance of paying greater attention to individual perceptions of support and there also appeared to be scope for reducing the deterioration in functioning by increasing social ties and participation. There was little scope for doing this by improving general practitioners' awareness and treatment of impairment. Most disabling symptoms had already been reported to doctors and many were being treated but the restriction of activity could have been reduced by the provision of aids and services. In addition, some of the symptoms associated with disability appeared to be the side effects of drugs and this pointed to a need for further studies of the potential for reducing the iatrogenic component of disability. Analyses of respondent satisfaction with medical care showed that those with disability tended to be more dissatisfied with their own doctors than those without disability, although the overall level of satisfaction in each group was high. The main area of dissatisfaction for both groups was the amount of information their own doctor had given them about their health.[169, 170]

Social and Economic Consequences of Disability

In order to have a more complete picture of the impact of chronic illness on everyday life in particular, life changes in general and people's methods of coping, a structured questionnaire was applied to a group of 24 people who were severely disabled by rheumatoid arthritis and whose disability was not of recent origin.[171] Each of the participants was interviewed twice in his or her own home and both interviews were tape recorded. The first interview was based on a common schedule of topic headings and probes, and was designed to cover as wide a range of their experiences as possible. The second interview, conducted one year later, was based on a similar schedule modified to take account of what each had said at the first interview that focused on changes in impairment, disability and personal circumstances. There was considerable variation in the problems experienced and the type of additional resources required by those who were limited in similar ways, reflecting differences in individual circumstances, knowledge and social skills. Some people, for example, were able to continue in employment because of the assistance of others, or the reorganisation of work, while others in less favourable environments became unemployed. Similarly, resources, in terms of money and appropriate physical environments, formed key factors in reflecting independent living.

Although this was a small study, and one cannot generalise from it, we found that the most disadvantaged did not appear to be overwhelmingly concentrated among the lower social economic groups. Opportunities for remaining in work, after the onset of disability, were not, for example, markedly different for those in a manual or non-manual occupation and the presence of supportive social networks was not confined to individuals in one particular social class.

Method for Assessing Preferences for Cash or Services

The Department of Health requested that the St Thomas' Unit develop methods for eliciting the preferences of disabled people for cash or services. Three methods were designed and tested on 305 disabled respondents and 59 carers. The services investigated were the home help service and a hypothetical visiting service. These services were selected as being ones for which lay substitutes were available. The hypothetical service was included to ascertain how respondents coped in assessing a service of which they have no experience. The amount of cash offered to each respondent was set at £2 per hour and the maximum number of hours offered was five. The methods tested were as follows:

1. Evaluation/trade-off in which respondents were asked what amount of money they would be prepared to pay for different numbers of hours of services.
2. Paired comparisons in which respondents were offered combinations of cash and services.
3. Budget allocation in which respondents were asked to use a decreasing number of vouchers to obtain home help, meals on wheels and home visiting in whatever combination they preferred and retain any number of vouchers as a cash limit.

The second method did not appear to be suitable for assessing preferences because of the time required for its administration and because the combination seemed unrealistic. Respondents found no difficulty with the other two methods, indicating that these could be more widely used. The results showed that the respondents who took cash were characterised by an unwillingness to accept the services offered. This suggests that the cash was preferred to indicate a lack of preference of services, rather than a specific preference for increased income.[172]

INFORMATION AND RESOURCE ALLOCATION

Towards the end of the 1960s concern began to be raised on the uneven distribution of resources for health care. MPs from the northern parts of the country, in their travels to and from their constituencies, noticed that new hospitals were being built in the South, but not the North. New hospital building only began in the 1960s, after the publication of a report on hospital building needs in 1962, while Enoch Powell was Minister of Health.[173] Between 1939 and the mid-1960s the only new hospital built in England was the Harvard Hospital on Salisbury Plain for US servicemen. Construction resources were required more urgently for house building to repair the ravages of Second World War bombing. The British Medical Association was also active in seeking medical resources – it was apparent to them that the budgets, staffing and equipment in the southern parts of England were greater than in the North.

Crossman, Secretary of State for Health and Social Security (1968–1970), responded to the political and professional pressure about unequal resources by examining the way in which resources were being distributed. The basis of allocation to each entity, region or Board of Governors was the amount of money they received in 1948 (the start of the NHS) plus a percentage increase each year, dependent on the general economic position and individual advocacy. Persuasive arguments by an authority resulted in a slightly greater proportionate increase than the general level. The level of funding had been unequal at the start of the NHS, when the richer parts of the country had higher levels of funding than the more deprived areas and so the differences between the various regions widened over time. In 1976–1977 there was an almost 30 per cent difference in the revenue allocation between the 14 regions per head of population, with the North West areas of the country having the least and North-East Thames region the most.[174] Differences in capital allocation were similar. As a result of this inequality of funding, a formula based on objective criteria was introduced to guide the distribution of hospital revenue to Regional Hospital Boards. This was known as the Crossman Formula although it was actually implemented by Sir Keith Joseph. The formula was based on three factors – population, beds and cases. The population factor was given an arbitrary double weight so that the relative contribution to the 'target' of the three elements was population 0.5, beds 0.25 and cases 0.25.[175] This is not the place to describe all the ramifications of the process of resource redistribution. Suffice it to say that the Crossman Formula was rapidly shown to be inadequate and a full account of this can be found in a paper by Mays and Bevan.[176] The fundamental problem was that the formula included a major contribution based on utilisation and current resources and since utilisation depends on availability of resources which were unequally distributed it could not rectify the problem.

When the Labour Party returned to power in 1974, with Barbara Castle as Secretary of State for Health, the problem of regional resource inequality was addressed again to modify the Crossman Formula. Professor Brian Abel Smith was a Special Adviser to the Secretary of State for Health with a particular interest in this problem (on which he had already advised Crossman, whose Special Adviser he had been earlier). He also chaired the Advisory Committee to the Social Medicine and Health Services Research Unit at St Thomas' and at a meeting of the Advisory Committee he drew attention to the problems of resource allocation and encouraged the Unit to consider possible research to rectify this unacceptable situation. As a result of this, a short draft proposal was developed. This suggested the Health Authorities should be classified into groups based on a number of criteria – total mortality, cardiovascular disease mortality, cancer mortality and perinatal mortality. Each group was to be divided, at random, into high or low mortality. In addition a number of Health Authorities were to be divided, at random, into two groups. Additional resources were then to be allocated to one of the groups with high total mortality, with no earmarking. Earmarked funds for cardiovascular services were to be given to half of the Health Authorities with high cardiovascular mortality, similarly to those with high cancer mortality and high perinatal mortality. Furthermore the Health Authorities not included among those classified as having a high cancer, cardiovascular or perinatal rate of mortality were divided into two groups, one to receive extra resources, the other not. It was thus envisaged that this complicated randomised controlled trial would answer three questions.

1.   Did additional resources improve health (to be measured by a variety of indices such as health care utilisation, mortality and random sample surveys of levels of function)?
2.   Did additional resources earmarked for certain services, such as maternity and child health, improve the health of mothers and children, as measured by perinatal and maternal mortality?
3.   Were earmarked increases in funding more effective than a non-specific general increase?

The proposal was sent to the Chief Scientist who considered that it was a feasible and interesting proposal which would need detailed work before it could be applied. As the proposal required a great deal of commitment from Health Authorities, the Chief Scientist also sent it to the Minister of Health, Dr David Owen, who invited myself, as the St Thomas' Unit Director, and the Chief Scientist to a meeting. He told us that the proposal was interesting but politically impossible. He could not envisage allocating resources to Health Authorities according to a random scheme and knew the idea would be savaged in the House of Commons. Owen was, however, very concerned to develop a more just and transparent scheme of resource allocation. He was about to convene a Working Party, the Resource Allocation Working Party (RAWP), to examine the possibilities and I was invited to become a member of the main group as well as its revenue and teaching and research subgroups. In view of the major time commitments entailed I was allowed to nominate a deputy to the revenue subgroup (Professor A.E. Bennett, who had been Deputy Director of the Social Medicine and Health Services Research Unit) and the teaching and research subgroup (Dr A.H. Snaith, Area Medical Officer, Avon Health Authority (Teaching), who had collaborated on several Unit research projects).

Membership of the RAWP led to a number of scientific publications,[175–183] but more importantly, the Unit prepared analyses of a variety of regional mortality and morbidity indicators for consideration of linking the allocation of resources to health needs. The Unit representatives were able to advise the RAWP on the reliability of the various indicators, their independence from available facilities and their association with health care needs. This advice helped in coming to the decision that the Standardised Mortality Ratios (SMR) were a reasonable indicator of regional variations in health care needs in the acute sector. The arguments against the use of other indicators and the methods used in the derivation of an appropriate formula for the allocation of resources are detailed in the final Report of the RAWP.[174]

The conclusions were the subject of some criticism from a variety of academic and operational research sources, as well as both departmental and regional/area administrators and finance officers. The review by Mays and Bevan in 1987 considered these, and concluded that the formula devised was reasonable:[176] 'RAWP, in most respects possessed remarkable soundness of judgement in its choice of information, boldness in conception, and grasp of the underlying objective and how in practice this might best be achieved' (p. 147). (It must be noted that Mays and Bevan were not in the Department or Unit at the time or involved in any way in the work.)

An important caveat was included in the conclusions of the Report by the RAWP, at the insistence of the Unit:[174]

> the prevalence of many of the conditions which are among the main causes of mortality is probably not significantly influenced by the intervention of health care services and that the redistribution of resources may not therefore have a significant and early impact on morbidity characteristics. But this cannot be a reason for ignoring them, since the NHS has a statutory responsibility to respond to the needs which those characteristics generate.

The Report[174] continued by emphasising the need to develop and apply: 'positive preventive measures (for example, by promoting changes in smoking habits) and by encouraging improvements in the environment in which people live and work' (pp. 84–5).

What Happened Later?

The formula devised by the RAWP, based on the work of a HSR Unit, with strong emphasis on epidemiology, was subject to a great deal of comment and criticism.

It was welcomed by the Northern regions, such as Trent, which gained resources at the expense of the Metropolitan regions. The most vicious opposition was from finance officers, those working in the Department of Health as well as regional officers. At the Department of Health there was a small unit of finance officers who were particularly upset. Since 1948 these individuals had been responsible for the allocation of resources between regions and Boards of Governors. For the first time all their power had been removed – distribution was now to occur based on challengeable, transparent data and simple principles. Regional Board Finance Officers were equally threatened – their decisions could now be challenged. The losing regions, particularly the four Metropolitan Thames regions, were extremely unhappy, as were most of the London Teaching Hospitals. Certainly the researchers at the St Thomas' Unit were not popular!

Politicians were also unhappy. Allocation to local government was and still is made on a complicated formula basis which takes into account such factors as proportion of ethnic minority groups, density of housing and so on. It was well known by civil servants that the formula was manipulated by each administration so that when Labour was in power, urban authorities gained, while rural areas gained when there was a Conservative administration. This was discussed by the RAWP and the decision not to include any 'deprivation' weighting in the formula but to use the SMR as the only factor, other than population–age–size, was because these figures could not be manipulated (if deprivation indices had been included there would, of course, have been double counting as the SMR is greatly affected by poverty).

The fact that no weighting factor was used was also attacked by operational researchers and economists who questioned that there was a one-to-one relationship between the SMR and the need for health services and wanted more elaborate models to be developed. Most epidemiologists questioned that need – their view was that, unless there was an underlying hypothesis, it was safer to use no weighting factor.

The concept that the SMR – that is, mortality – could be used to influence the distribution of health resources was also questioned by many on the grounds that much health care is provided for individuals who do not die – for example, those undergoing hernia or hip operations. They neglected to take into account that there is little geographical variation in these conditions in contrast to, for example, cancer and cardiovascular disease.

In spite of these considerations the formula devised by the RAWP was applied until 1989. It was successful in reducing the gap between the resources of the Northern and the Metropolitan regions. The narrowing of this gap was achieved more rapidly than expected, largely because there was a decline in the total resources of the NHS.

Political pressure increased considerably, particularly from the more affluent regions, and so a Review was set up. The major criticisms to be addressed were threefold: (1) measures of morbidity, since the SMR was not considered a good proxy; (2) that the SMR did not capture the full consequences of social and economic deprivation; and (3) that there was no empirical reason for the one-to-one relationship between the SMR and need for health care resources.

The Review proposed that need for health care should be based on a model derived from small area statistics rather than relying on one outcome measure (mortality).[184, 185] This model would take account of variations in hospital utilisation adjusted for the supply of facilities accessible to the area and such factors as age–sex distribution, population size and social class. The Review team also suggested replacing the all-age SMR with the SMR <75 together with a reduction of the weighting given to the SMR in the formula from 1.0 to 0.44 and the inclusion of the Jarman deprivation score (a score based on the opinions of a number of GPs of the factors affecting need for health services), both to be weighted in accordance with their estimated coefficients from the regression analysis. Ministers decided not to include the Jarman score and to weight the SMR with an elasticity of 0.5.[186] This was announced with the publication of *Working for Patients* in 1989.[187]

None of the original members of the RAWP were involved or consulted. Much of the technical work was carried out by a management consultancy firm, Coopers and Lybrand. This formula was subjected to criticism for its conceptualisation of need (use of utilisation data with inadequate consideration of supply effects), adequacy of the database used (only six out of 14 regions) and the appropriateness of the statistical measures used.[188, 189]

Further concern with the formula for resource allocation has continued. An interesting contribution to the debate was made by a group of geographers and sociologists from Plymouth.[190] In an analysis of coronary heart disease in 34 Primary Care Trusts they appeared to demonstrate that moving to a morbidity-based model would result in a significant shift in hospital resources away from deprived areas towards areas with older demographic profiles and towards rural areas.

In view of the changes in NHS structure it is not surprising that another major report was published in 2008.[191] This recommended major changes, the most significant being that post 2010/11 GP registered lists should be used, that age and additional need are calculated in a single index based on admitted patient and outpatient data, that there should be a separate formula for health inequalities and that the market forces factor should be refined. Most recently, a team from the Nuffield Trust has suggested further changes based on complex models of need for individual practices; need being equated to utilisation with a variety of adjustments for supply.[192]

The original formula developed for resource allocation by the RAWP was relatively simple and based on pragmatic principles of transparency and comprehensibility. It offended a variety of interest groups, politicians, operational researchers and economists with its simplicity. With innumerable changes in NHS organisation and structure, the availability of much more patient data, and the increasing influence of economists in influencing NHS decisions, the formula has changed considerably. It is now complex, highly dependent on a series of statistical assumptions of unproven reliability, and far less dependent on epidemiological principles. The original formula did achieve a significant redistribution of resources. It is difficult to determine whether the 'fiddles' which the RAWP eschewed have achieved their objectives.

AVOIDABLE DEATHS

In the early 1980s the NHS and the Department of Health began to be concerned with the measurement and assessment of health services' performance. A variety of financial measures were being proposed and used, such as programme budgeting and keeping to budget. In addition the media made much play of waiting lists and this has continued. A number of studies were also published on geographical variation in the frequency with which various procedures, such as hysterectomy, were being carried out. The earliest work in this field can probably be traced to Glover in 1938, a school medical officer who noted the wide variation in the incidence of tonsillectomy undertaken in children of the same age in different schools.[193] Glover could not find any reason for the variation in tonsillectomy other than custom. This work was further developed by Wennberg and Gittelsohn in 1973, who showed unexplained (and unwarranted) small area variations in the rates for common procedures based on Medicare data for the elderly in the US.[194]

Variations in the number of procedures undertaken in different populations are examples of process measures that may illuminate the performance of health services. These process measures are easily obtained and are popular with administrators, politicians and others; but because they do not measure outcome, they do not address the essential function of health services.

In the nineteenth century, Florence Nightingale put forward the concept of hospital mortality. The difficulty with this as a measure of performance is that the patients treated in different hospitals vary in regard to many characteristics so that it is difficult to draw any valid conclusions. It was nonetheless an outstanding achievement. Codman, a US surgeon (1869–1940), attempted to document hospital surgical outcomes and published all errors – 123 in 337 patients.[195] Paul Lembcke, an epidemiologist at Johns Hopkins University School of Hygiene, Baltimore, Maryland, reintroduced the concept of looking at the outcomes of hospital care and related it to defined geographical populations.[196] Unfortunately none of these studies were pursued by those involved in the assessment of health service performance. Various arguments were used to dismiss these measures, principally, the problem of case-mix – that is, variations in age–sex distribution and in different conditions and their severity.

As an epidemiologist, I did not consider that a process measure was an adequate tool for the ultimate aim of assessment of health service delivery. In 1984–1985 I had the opportunity of spending time at the US National Institute of Health in Bethesda, Maryland, as a Fogarty Scholar-in-Residence. I used this opportunity to try to identify suitable measures for the assessment of health service outcome, at population level, by visiting and talking to a number of leading workers in the field as well as a comprehensive search of published literature. I was fortunate to have access to the computerised databases of health literature at the US National Library of Medicine. In the literature, there were remarkably few examples of measures capable of assessing outcomes for populations that could be used as a routine measure on a population level. The only publications that I could find among the many thousands that I searched were the two publications by the Rutstein Working Group.[197, 198]

The Rutstein Group examined the causes of death and decided which ones could be used as 'quality of care' indices. The aim was to identify a series of indicators of avoidable disease, disability and death – that is, sentinel adverse health events. They assumed that if everything had gone well, the condition would have been prevented or managed successfully. Of course, they realised that the chain of responsibility was very long, making it difficult to identify who was actually responsible for any treatment or system failure. The conditions chosen were divided into three different types. First came those that were clear-cut and could be used as immediate quality of care indices, consisting of over 100 conditions further divided into unnecessary disease, unnecessary disability and unnecessary, untimely death. The majority of conditions in this category were infectious diseases such as measles, rubella and yellow fever. There were also a number of chronic conditions including some cancers, such as neoplasms of the cervix, lung and trachea, gout, hypervitaminosis, glaucoma and infections of the skin. The second group of conditions were those considered to be of limited use as indicators of quality of care and included bacillary dysentery, food poisoning and haemophilia. Third were conditions that required better definition and special studies before their relationship with quality of care could be determined.

The difficulty with this classification was that it was far too wide and there was little consideration of the factors or interventions that could have prevented untimely death. Little attempt had been made to identify what practicable interventions would have been feasible and thus the classification was too vague for use in practice. Remarkably it was never applied in the US in the assessment of quality of health services in spite of two of the many authors being Dr Tom Chalmers, Medical Director of the Veterans Administration, and Professor Ed Perrin, Director of the US National Center for Health Statistics. Possibly they acknowledged its inadequacy but considered that it should be used to stimulate further, more precise development.

I considered that this classification could be useful in the measurement of NHS performance. A simpler method of classification, restricted to 14 causes of death in clearly specified age–sex ranges, was developed. This identified the major health care providers involved in the care of these conditions and the aspect of health care that could potentially influence mortality. A paper was published in the *Lancet* in 1983 which showed variations of up to six-fold in the mortality of the chosen conditions by Area Health Authority.[199] The mortality rates were adjusted by age – that is, published as SMR. Deliberately, no adjustment for differences in deprivation in the different areas was made. This led to some comment but we maintained that there was no reason why the services provided in the more deprived areas should be any worse than in the more affluent areas. Furthermore, health services were supposed to react to need – so areas with a higher incidence of a particular disease ought to adapt to the greater need for treatment for this condition. The publication aroused a great deal of interest in the media. *The Sunday Times* published an atlas of avoidable mortality based on our work and there were some TV programmes on services in the worst areas, in which these areas naturally defended their records vehemently[200]. Care had been taken, before publication, to discuss the findings with the Regional Medical Officers. It was interesting that none questioned our findings, and in one region the Regional Medical Officer congratulated us and stated that 'at last' confirmation of the inadequacy of health services in one affluent area had been provided. For each condition, the services important in preventing mortality were identified.[201] The findings of the analysis were interesting. Some of the areas with the lowest rates of avoidable mortality were in the North-East, an area with a good reputation for its health services. Another area with low avoidable mortality was Sheffield. Thus areas with high levels of poverty could excel in the quality of health services provided. By contrast high levels of mortality were occurring in parts of the West Midlands and the North West – with wealthier areas having a better record than those in the poorer areas. Areas with high levels of avoidable mortality were encouraged to undertake confidential enquiries in order to try to identify the causes of high mortality. These enquiries were conducted by local clinicians and we provided some methodological assistance. The local clinicians laid down criteria of what care should have been received, in their view and in their circumstances, by the patients who had died from one of the conditions. This local investigation was deliberate since it was hoped that the identification of failures by those responsible for delivering the service was the most likely way to improve the quality of health care in the area.

The model for these confidential enquiries was the model pioneered by the Confidential Enquiry into Maternal Deaths.[202, 203] These enquiries, for example, showed that in one area, while patients with hypertension had been referred and investigated critically and adequately by the appropriate specialist service, they had not been referred back to their general practitioner but were 'retained' in outpatients. Over time the individual grade of clinician examining the patient became more junior and less experienced and treatment became inadequate. An appropriate change in the handling of this type of patient was introduced. In another area patients dying from cervical cancer had been screened appropriately but the findings of the cervical smear test were retained in the laboratory instead of being reported to the patient's GP so that no treatment was instituted. In another region far too few patients were screened for cervical cancer because of inadequate cervical screening services. In both the last two examples the service deficiencies were rectified and some seven years later the cervical cancer mortality rate had been reduced.

These investigations of avoidable mortality were used for a large number of national and international comparisons of health service performance and led to a number of cooperative studies in the European Community as well as elsewhere.[204-212] These and other studies have been reviewed more recently.[213] The European Community has in 2009–2012 funded a major cooperative research effort, led by Professors McKee and Mackenbach, to update this research and explore further uses (AMIEHS).[ii]

Unfortunately, although this relatively simple measure to assess the quality and performance of clinical care has aroused a great deal of activity among academics, relatively few health authorities have applied it to the active improvement of care. Clinicians have, however, applied the concept enthusiastically – for example, obstetricians in influencing maternity care, and surgeons and physicians in examining a variety of procedures.

CONCLUSION

The intention in this chapter has been to provide examples of HSR undertaken by the St Thomas' Research Unit between 1962 and 1994. The reasons behind the particular projects and the findings have been described.

The research covered many areas of relevance to the delivery of health services and the maintenance and promotion of health. They included: studies of the provision of health care services in a given population (Lambeth, Basingstoke and Frimley); studies of individual services such as multiphasic screening, examination of an individual procedure (lithotripsy); and investigations of specific disciplines such as general practice and psychiatry. There were also epidemiological investigations: of methods to deter smoking and reduce the harm of smoking: of the maintenance of a national system of surveillance of nutrition to assess the effect of a decision to change welfare policy; and of the development and use of a performance measure (avoidable death), nationally and internationally.

It is striking that at the beginning of its work, the Unit was encouraged to become involved in studies of the organisation of the service provided for a defined population in the areas mentioned above. In the later period, research tended to be confined largely to research on specific services or aspects of the Health Service. As the Unit was led by an epidemiologist, most of the studies followed the proven principles of that discipline – the

---

ii AMIEHS – Avoidable Mortality in the European Union. Towards better Indicators for the Effectiveness of Health Services.

collection of original data – although every study also involved other disciplines. In contrast to more recent examples of HSR, the Unit was determined to use and if necessary collect the data appropriate to answer a specific question rather than being dependent on large data-sets collected for a different, more universal purpose or for administrative use.

The studies illustrate the wide variety of research designs used and the need for the development and application of specific instruments. Failures are included as well as successful studies in the hope of providing evidence of the prerequisites of worthwhile research. That a piece of research is successfully implemented and applied, often for a limited time only, is perhaps inevitable. But it does underline the fundamental importance of being aware of and if necessary able to apply historical findings as well as new research.

That HSR and its results are a highly emotive political subject must never be forgotten. The changes in resource allocation within the NHS demonstrate how methods of policy implementation can be affected with no change in the underlying facts but with changes in political administration and the influence of particular interest groups. Similarly, findings of consequence – for example, initial evidence of childhood obesity – may be dismissed or neglected, with serious consequences, because they threaten industrial or commercial interests.

Although the research described was undertaken by one Unit, these studies illustrate the ways in which rigorous HSR can help to improve health and health care delivery.

REFERENCES

1 Clarke, M., Waller, J. and Webster, B. (1975). The assessment and progress of long-stay and elderly psychiatric patients; the predictive validity of a ward behaviour questionnaire. *British Journal of Psychiatry*, **127**, 149–56.
2 Clarke, M. and Waller, J. (1974). Descriptive studies of a psychiatric hospital population. *British Journal of Psychiatry*, **125**, 208–9.
3 Adler, M.W., Waller, J.J., Day, I., Kasap, H.S. and Thorne, S.C. (1978). Randomised controlled trial of discharge for inguinal hernia. *Journal of Epidemiology and Community Health*, **32**, 136–42.
4 Trevelyan, M.H. and Cook, J. (1974). The use of acute medical and general-practitioner beds by the practitioners working in one new town. *Journal of the Royal College of General Practitioners*, **2**, 477–87.
5 Weddell, J.M. and Beresford, S.A.A. (1979). *Planning for Stroke Patients: a Four-year Descriptive Study of Home and Hospital Care.* London: HMSO.
6 Cochrane, A.L. (1971). *Random Reflections on Health Services.* Rock Carling Fellowship. London: Nuffield Provincial Hospitals Trust.

7 Rothschild Report (1971). The organisation and management of Government R&D. In: *Cabinet Office: A Framework for Government Research and Development*. London: HMSO.

8 McLachlan, G. (ed.) (1971), *Portfolio for Health 1. The Role and Programme of the DHSS in Health Services Research. Problems and Progress in Medical Care. 6th Series. Essays on Current Research*. London: Oxford University Press for the Nuffield Provincial Hospitals Trust.

9 Holland, W.W. and Gilderdale, S. (1973). Evaluating Need and Demand. In: *New Concepts of Management in the NHS: a Report of a Seminar*. The Royal College of General Practitioners, Merseyside and N. Wales Faculty. RCGP: 22-30, 13 May.

10 Holland, W.W. and Waller, J.J. (1971). Population studies in the London Borough of Lambeth. *Community Medicine*, **126**, 153–6.

11 Bennett, A.E. and Kasap, H.S. (1970). Data processing for a private census. In: Holland, W.W. (ed.), *Data Handling in Epidemiology*. London: Oxford University Press, pp. 11–124.

12 Palmer, J.W., Kasap, H.S., Bennett, A.E. and Holland, W.W. (1969). The use of hospitals by a defined population. A community and hospital study in North Lambeth. *British Journal of Preventive and Social Medicine*, **23**(2), 91–100.

13 Garrod, J, and Bennett, A.E. (1971). A validated interview schedule for use in population surveys of chronic disease and disability. *British Journal of Preventive and Social Medicine*, **25**, 97–104.

14 Bennett, A.E., Garrod, J. and Halil, T. (1970). Chronic disease and disability in the community: a prevalence study. *British Medical Journal*, **ii**, 762–4.

15 Raftery, E.B., Cocker, P. and Holland, W.W. (1971). The value of the electrocardiogram in population survey: an attempt to improve interpretation. *British Heart Journal*, **33**, 837–40.

16 Adler, M.W., Illiffe, J.L., Holland, W.W. and Kasap, H.S. (1973). Assessment of medical care needs of individuals with chronic cardio-respiratory disease using subjection measures. *International Journal of Epidemiology*, **2**, 73–9.

17 Rea, J.N., Newhouse, M.L. and Halil, T. (1976). Skin diseases in Lambeth: a community study of prevalence and use of medical care. *British Journal of Preventive and Social Medicine*, **30**, 107–14.

18 Clarke, M., Halil, T. and Salmon, N. (1976). Peptic ulceration in men: epidemiology and medical care. *British Journal of Preventive and Social Medicine*, **30**, 115–22.

19 Adler, M.W., Waller, J.J., Day, I., Kasap, H.S., King, C. and Thorne, S.C. (1974). A randomised controlled trial of early discharge for inguinal hernia and varicose veins: some problems of methodology. *Medical Care*, **12**, 541–7.

20 Adler, M.W. (1977). *A Randomised Controlled Trial of Early Discharge for Inguinal Hernia and Varicose Veins*. MD Thesis. University of London.

21 Adler, M.W. (1977). Randomised controlled trial of early discharge for inguinal hernia and varicose veins. *Annals of the Royal College of Surgeons of England*, **59**, 251–4.

22 Adler, M.W. (1978). Changes in local clinical practice following an experiment in medical care: evaluation of evaluation. *Journal of Epidemiology and Community Health*, **32**, 143–6.

23 Waller, J.J., Adler, M.W., Creese, A.L. and Thorne, S.C. (1978). *Early Discharge from Hospital for Patients with Hernia or Varicose Veins. A Report of a Randomised Controlled Trial*. London: HMSO.

24 Clarke, M. and Mulholland, A. (1973). The use of general practitioner beds. *Journal of the Royal College of General Practitioners*, **23**, 273–9.

25 Holland, W.W. and Stewart, S. (1990). *Screening in Health Care. Benefit or Bane?* London: Nuffield Provincial Hospitals Trust.

26 Holland, W.W. and Stewart, S. (2005). *Screening in Disease Prevention. What Works?* Oxford: Radcliffe Publishing for Nuffield Trust and European Observatory on Health Systems and Policies.

27 Holland, W.W. (2009). Periodic Health Examination – a brief history and critical assessment. *Eurohealth*, **15**, 16–20.

28 Wilson, J.M.G and Jungner, G. (1968). *Principles and Practice of Screening for Disease*. Geneva: World Health Organisation.

29 South East London Screening Study Group (1977). A controlled trial of multiphasic screening in middle-age: results of the South East London Screening Study. *International Journal of Epidemiology*, **6**, 357–63.

30 D'Souza. M.F., Swan, A.V. and Shannon, D.J. (1976). A long-term controlled trial of screening for hypertension in general practice. *Lancet*, **1**, 1228–31.

31 D'Souza, M.F. (1978). Early diagnosis and multiphasic screening. In: Bennett, A.E. (ed.), *Recent Advances in Community Medicine*. Edinburgh: Churchill Livingstone, pp. 195–214.

32 D'Souza, M.F. (1979). *General Health Screening: an Assessment of its Value in Middle-age*. MD Thesis, University of London.

33 Trevelyan, M.H. (1973). Study to evaluate the effects of multiphasic screening within general practice in Britain. Design and method. *Preventive Medicine*, **1**, 278–94.

34 Holland, W.W. and Whitehead, T.P. (1974). Value of new laboratory tests in diagnosis and treatment. *Lancet*, **2**(7895), 1494–7.

35 Whitehead, T.P. (1973). The Wolfson Research Laboratories. In: McLachlan, G. (ed.), *Portfolio for Health 2: The Developing Programme of the DHSS in Health Services Research. Problems and Progress in Medical Care. 8th Series. Essays on Current Research*. London: Oxford University Press for the Nuffield Provincial Hospitals Trust, pp. 143–9.

36 Mays, N., Challah, S., Patel, S., Palfrey, E., Creese, A., Vadera, P. and Burney, P. (1988). Clinical comparison of extra-corporeal shock wave lithotripsy with percutaneous surgery in the treatment of renal calculi. *British Medical Journal*, **297**, 253–8.

37 Mays, N., Petruckevitch, A. and Burney, P.G.J. (1992). Results of one and two year follow-up of a clinical comparison of extra-corporeal shock wave lithotripsy and percutaneous nephrolithotomy in the treatment of renal calculi. *Scandinavian Journal of Urology and Nephrology*, **26**, 43–9.

38 Mays, N. (1991). Relative costs and cost-effectivenesss of extra-corporeal shock wave lithotripsy versus percutaneous nephrolithotomy in the treatment of renal and ureteric stones. *Social Science and Medicine*, **32**, 1401–12.
39 Mays, N., Petruckevitch, A. and Snowden, C. (1990). Patient's quality of life following extra-corporeal shock wave lithotripsy and percutaneous nephrolithotomy for renal calculi. *International Journal of Technology Assessment in Health Care*, **6**, 633–2.
40 Rona, R.J., Swan, A.V., Beech, R., Prentice, L., Reynolds, A., Wilson, O., Mole, G. and Vadera, P. (1989). Demand for DNA probe testing in three genetic centres in Britain (August 1986 –July 1987). *Journal of Medical Genetics*, **26**, 226–36.
41 Beech, R., Rona, R.J., Swan, A.V., Kavanagh, F.B., Prentice, L., Wilson, O.M., Mole, G. and Vadera, P. (1989). Genetic services in the context of DNA probes: what do they cost? *Journal of Medical Genetics*, **26**, 237–44.
42 Rona, R.J., Swan, A.V., Beech, R., Wilson, O.M., Kavanagh, F.B., Brown, C., Axtell, C. and Mandalia, S. (1992). DNA probe technology: implications for service planning in Britain. *Clinical Genetics*, **42**, 186–95.
43 Beech, R., Rona, R.J., Swan, A.V., Wilson, O.M. and Mandalia, S. (1992). A methodology for simulating the impact of DNA probe services on the outcome of pregnancies. *International Journal of Technology Assessment in Health Care*, **8**, 539–45.
44 Rona, R.J. and Beech, R. (1993). The process of evaluation of a new technology: genetic services and the introduction of DNA probes. *Journal of Public Health Medicine*, **15**, 185–91.
45 Colley, J.R.T and Holland, W.W. (1967). Social and environmental factors in respiratory diseases. A preliminary report. *Archives of Environmental Health*, **14**, 157–61.
46 Holland, W.W., Kasap, H.S., Colley, J.T.R. and Cormack, W. (1969). Respiratory symptoms and ventilatory function: a family study. *British Journal of Preventive and Social Medicine*, **23**, 77–84.
47 Collins, J.J., Kasap, H.S. and Holland, W.W. (1971). Environmental factors in child mortality in England and Wales. *American Journal of Epidemiology*, **93**, 10–22.
48 Holland, W.W. and Elliott, A. (1968). Cigarette Smoking, respiratory symptoms and anti-smoking propaganda. *Lancet*, **1**, 41–3.
49 Holland, W.W., Halil, T., Bennett, A.E. and Elliott, A. (1969). Factors influencing the onset of chronic respiratory disease. *British Medical Journal*, **2**, 205–8.
50 Holland, W.W., Halil, T., Bennett, A.E. and Elliott, A. (1969). Indications for measures to be taken in childhood to prevent chronic respiratory disease. *Milbank Memorial Fund Quarterly*, **47**, 215–27.
51 Holland, W.W., Halil, T. and Elliott, A. (1969). The effect of environmental factors on ventilatory function in schoolchildren. In: Proceedings of the 11th Aspen Emphysema Conference, Aspen, CO, June 12–15, 1968, Arlington, VA: USDHEW, pp. 259–72.
52 Holland, W.W., Halil, T., Bennett, A.E. and Elliott, A. (1970). Estimating the influence of personal and environmental factors on ventilatory function

and respiratory symptoms. In: Orie, N.G.M. and van der Lende, R. (eds), *Bronchitis III, Proceedings of the Third International Symposium on Bronchitis, Groningen, 23–26 September 1969*. Assen. Royal Vangorcum, pp. 20–30.

53 Bennett, A.E., Holland, W.W., Halil, T. and Elliott, A. (1971). Lung function and air pollution. In: Ulmer, W.T. (ed.), Chronic inflammation of the bronchi. *Progress in Respiratory Research*, **6**, 78–89.

54 Colley, J.R.T., Holland, W.W. and Corkhill, R.T. (1974). Influence of passive smoking and parental phlegm on pneumonia and bronchitis in childhood. *Lancet*, **2**, 1031–4.

55 Leeder, S.R., Corkhill, R.T., Irwig, L.M., Holland, W.W. and Colley, J.R.T. (1976). Influence of family factors on asthma and wheezing during the first five years of life. *British Journal of Preventive and Social Medicine*, **30**, 213–18.

56 Leeder, S.R., Corkhill, R.T., Irwig, L.M., Holland, W.W. and Colley, J.R.T. (1976). Influence of family factors on the incidence of lower respiratory illness during the first year of life. *British Journal of Preventive and Social Medicine*, **30**, 203–12.

57 Leeder, S.R., Corkhill, R.T., Wysocki, M.J., Holland, W.W. and Colley, J.R.T. (1976). Influence of personal and family factors on ventilatory function of children. *British Journal of Preventive and Social Medicine*, **30**, 219–24.

58 Bland, J.M., Holland, W.W. and Elliott. A. (1974). The development of respiratory symptoms in a cohort of Kent schoolchildren. *Bulletin de Physiopathologie Respiratoire*, **10**, 699–716.

59 Colley, J.R.T., Holland, W.W., Leeder, S.R. and Corkhill, R.T. (1976). Respiratory function of infants in relation to subsequent respiratory disease. An epidemiological study. *Bulletin de Physiopathologie Respiratoire*, **12**, 651–7.

60 Bland, J.M., Bewley, B.R., Pollard, V. and Banks, M.H. (1978). Effect of children's and parents' smoking on respiratory symptoms. *Archives of Disease in Childhood*, **53**, 100–105.

61 Holland, W.W., Bailey, P. and Bland, J.M. (1978). Long term consequences of respiratory diseases in infancy. *Journal of Epidemiology and Community Health*, **32**, 256–9.

62 Swan, A.V., Murray, M. and Jarrett, L. (1991). *Smoking Behaviour from Pre-Adolescence to Young Adulthood*. Aldershot: Avelbury, Gower Publishing.

63 Murray, M., Jarrett, L., Swan, A.V. and Rumun, R. (1988). *Smoking in Young Adults*. Aldershot: Avelbury, Gower Publishing.

64 Bewley, B.R. (1991). *Prevalence of Smoking in Final Year Primary Schoolchildren (Derbyshire) and some Associated Factors*. MSc Thesis, University of London.

65 Bewley, B.R., Halil, T. and Snaith, A. (1973). Smoking by primary schoolchildren: prevalence and associated respiratory symptoms. *British Journal of Preventive and Social Medicine*, **27**, 150–153.

66 Bewley, B.R., Bland, J.M. and Harris, R. (1974). Factors associated with the starting of cigarette smoking by primary schoolchildren. *British Journal of Preventive and Social Medicine*, **28**, 37–44.

67 Bland, J.M., Bewley, B.R., Banks, M.H. and Pollard, V. (1975). Schoolchildren's beliefs about smoking and disease. *Health Education Journal*, **34**, 71–8.

68 Bland, J.M., Bewley, B.R. and Day, I. (1975). Primary schoolboys: image of self and smoker. *British Journal of Preventive and Social Medicine*, **29**, 262–6.

69 Bewley, B.R. and Bland, J.M. (1976). Smoking and respiratory symptoms in two groups of schoolchildren. *Preventive Medicine*, **5**, 63–9.

70 Bewley, B.R. and Bland, J.M. (1977). Academic performance and social factors related to cigarette smoking by schoolchildren. *British Journal of Preventive and Social Medicine*, **31**, 18–24.

71 Banks, M.H., Bewley, B.P., Bland, J.M., Dean, J.R. and Pollard, V. (1978). Long-term study of smoking by secondary schoolchildren. *Archives of Disease in Childhood*, **53**, 12–19.

72 Bewley, B.R. (1978). The aims and objectives of health education in children. *SW Thames Regional Cancer Council Bulletin*, October.

73 Banks, M.H. (1979). *Social and Psychological Factors Involved in Adolescent Cigarette Smoking*. PhD Thesis, University of London.

74 Bewley, B.R., Johnson, M.R.D. and Banks, M.H. (1979). Teachers' smoking. *Journal of Epidemiology and Community Health*, **33**, 219–22.

75 Bewley, B.R., Johnson, M.R.D., Bland, J.M. and Murray, M. (1980). Trends in children's smoking. *Community Medicine*, **2**, 186–9.

76 Banks, M.H., Bewley, B.R. and Bland, J.M. (1981). Adolescent attitudes to smoking: their influence on behaviour. *International Journal of Health Education*, **14**, 39–44.

77 Johnson, M.R.D., Murray, M., Bewley, B.R., Clyde, D.C., Banks, M.H. and Swan, A.V. (1982). Social class, parents, children and smoking. *Bulletin International Union Against Tuberculosis*, **57**, 258–62.

78 Murray, M., Swan, A.V., Bewley, B.R. and Johnson, M.R.D. (1983). The development of smoking during adolescence: the MRC/Derbyshire Smoking Study. *International Journal of Epidemiology*, **12**, 185–92.

79 Murray, M., Swan, A.V., Johnson, M.R.D. and Bewley, B.R. (1983). Some factors associated with increased risk of smoking by children. *Journal of Child Psychology and Psychiatry*, **24**, 223–32.

80 Murray, M., Rona, R.J., Morris, R.W. and Tait, N. (1984). The smoking and dietary behaviours of Lambeth schoolchildren. I The effectiveness of an anti-smoking and nutrition education programme for children. *Public Health*, **98**, 163–72.

81 Murray, M., Swan, A.V. and Clarke, G. (1984). Long-term effect of a school-based anti-smoking programme. *Journal of Epidemiology and Community Health*, **38**, 247–52.

82 Murray, M., Kiryluk, S. and Swan, A.V. (1984). School characteristics and adolescent smoking. *Journal of Epidemiology and Community Health*, **38**, 167–72.

83 Murray, M. and Jarrett, L. (1985). Young people's perception of health and illness. *Health Education Journal,* **44**(1), 18–22.

84 Murray, M., Kiryluk, S. and Swan, A.V. (1985). Relation between parents' and children's smoking behaviour and attitudes. *Journal of Epidemiology and Community Health,* **39**, 169–74.

85 Johnson, M.R.D., Bewley, B.R., Banks, M.H., Bland, J.M. and Clyde, D.V. (1985). Smoking at school. *British Journal of Educational Psychology,* **55**, 35–44.

86 Independent Scientific Committee on Smoking and Health (1975). *First Report. Tobacco Substitutes and Additives in Tobacco Products.* London: HMSO.

87 Independent Scientific Committee on Smoking and Health (1979). *Second Report. Developments in Tobacco Products and the Possibility of Lower Risk Cigarettes.* London: HMSO.

88 Jarvis, M. and Russell, M.A.H. (1980). Comment on the Hunter Committee's second report. *British Medical Journal,* **280**, 994–5.

89 Swann, C. and Froggatt, P. (1996). *The Tobacco Products Research Trust.* London: Royal Society of Medicine Press.

90 Withey, C.H., Papacosta, A.O., Swann, A.V., Fitzsimons, A. Burney, P.G.J., Colley, J.R.T. and Holland, W.W. (1992). Respiratory effects of lowering tar and nicotine levels of cigarettes smoked by young male middle tar smokers. I Design of a randomised controlled trial. *Journal of Epidemiology and Community Health,* **46**, 274–80.

91 Withey, C.H., Papacosta, A.O., Swann, A.V., Fitzsimons, A. Burney, P.G.J., Colley, J.R.T. and Holland, W.W. (1992). Respiratory effects of lowering tar and nicotine levels of cigarettes smoked by young male middle tar smokers. II Results of a randomised controlled trial. *Journal of Epidemiology and Community Health,* **46**, 281–5.

92 Chinn, S., Britton, J.R., Burney, P.G.J., Tattersfield, A.E. and Papacosta, A.O. (1987). Estimations and repeatability of response to inhaled histamine in a community survey. *Thorax,* **42**, 45–52, 1987.

93 Burney, P.G.J., Britton, J.R., Chinn, S., Tattersfield, A.E., *et al.* (1987). The descriptive epidemiology of bronchial reactivity in an adult population: results from a community survey. *Thorax,* **42**, 38–44.

94 Chinn, S., Burney, P.G.J. (1987). On measuring repeatability of data for self-administered questionnaires. *International Journal of Epidemiology,* **16**, 121–7, 1987.

95 Burney, P.G.J. and Chinn, S. (1987). Developing a new questionnaire for measuring the prevalence of asthma. *Chest,* **97**, 79s–93s.

96 Burney, P.G.J. (1987). The causes of asthma – does salt potentiate bronchial activity. *Journal of the Royal Society of Medicine,* **80**, 364–7.

97 Britton, J.R., Chinn, S., Burney, P.G.J., Papacosta, A.O. and Tattersfield, A.E. (1988). Seasonal variation in bronchial reactivity in a community population. *Journal of Allergy and Clinical Immunology,* **82**, 134–9.

98 Britton, J.R., Burney, P.G.J., Chinn, S., Papacosta, A.O. and Tattersfield, A.E. (1988). The relation between change in airway reactivity and change in respiratory symptoms and medication in a community study. *American Review of Respiratory Disease,* **138**, 530–534.

99 Burney, P.G.J., Chinn, S., Britton, J.R., Tattersfield, A.E. and Papacosta, A.O. (1989). What symptoms predict the bronchial response to histamine? Evaluation of the IUATLD. Bronchial symptom questionnaire (1984) in a community survey. *International Journal of Epidemiology*, **18**, 165–73.

100 Burney, P.G.J., Laitinen, L., Perdrizet, S. *et al.* (1989). Validity and repeatability of the IUATLD (1984) bronchial symptom questionnaire: an international comparison. *European Respiratory Journal*, **2**, 940–945.

101 Burney, P.G.J., Britton, J.R., Chinn, S. *et al.* (1986). Response to inhaled histamine and 24 hour sodium excretion. *British Medical Journal*, **292**, 1483–6.

102 Burney, P.G.J., Papacosta, A.O., Withey, C.H., Colley, J.R.T. and Holland, W.W. (1991). Hospital admission rates and the prevalence of asthmatic symptoms in 20 local authority districts. *Thorax*, **46**, 574–9.

103 Burney, P.G.J. (1993). Evidence for an increase in atopic disease and possible causes. *Clinical and Experimental Allergy*, **23**, 484–92.

104 Chinn, S., Burney, P.G.J., Tattersfield, A.E. and Higgins, B.G. (1993). Comparison of PD20 with two alternative measures of response to histamine challenge in epidemiological studies. *European Respiratory Journal*, **6**, 670–679.

105 Higgins, B.G., Britton, J.R., Chinn, S., Lai, K.K. and Burney, P.G.J. (1993). Factors affecting peak expiratory flow variability and bronchial reactivity in a random population sample. *Thorax*, **48**, 899–905.

106 Luczynska, C.M., Bond, J. and Burney, P.G.J. (1993). A study of indoor allergen exposure and allergic disease in adults: an additional EC Respiratory Health Survey Protocol. *Allergy*, **48**, 1034.

107 Secretaries of State for Health and Social Security, Wales and Scotland (1989). *Caring for People: Community Care in the Next Decade and Beyond*. CMMD. 849. London: HMSO.

108 House of Commons Social Services Committee (1985). *Community Care with Special Reference to Adult Mentally Ill and Mentally Handicapped People*. Volume 1. HC13-I. London: HMSO.

109 Shepherd, M. (1966). *Psychiatric Illness in General Practice*. London: Oxford University Press.

110 Shepherd, M. (1980). Mental health as an integral of primary medical care. *Journal of the Royal College of General Practitioners*, **30**, 657–64.

111 Watts, C.A.H. (1966). *Depressive Disorders in the Community*. Bristol: John Wright.

112 Wing, J.K. and Hailey, A. (eds) (1972). *Evaluating a Community Psychiatric Service*. London: Oxford University Press for the Nuffield Provincial Hospitals Trust.

113 Wing, J.K. (1989). The measurement of 'social disablement'. The MRC social behaviour and social role performance schedules. *Social Psychiatry and Psychiatric Epidemiology*, **24**, 173–8.

114 Mezey, A.G., Hodkinson, H.M. and Evans, G.J. The elderly in the wrong unit. *British Medical Journal*, **3**, 16–18.

115 Player, D.A., Irving, G. and Robinson, R.A. (1971). Psychiatric, psychological and social findings in a pilot community health survey. *Health Bulletin*, **29**, 104–7.

116 Kushlick, A. (1971). *Epidemiological studies on and evaluation of services for the mentally subnormal and elderly*. Report to the MRC and DHSS, mimeographed. London: Medical Research Council.

117 Edwards, G. (1972). The development of the Addiction Research Unit of the Institute of Psychiatry, London. *Psychological Medicine*, **2**, 192–7.

118 Goldberg, D., Jackson, G., Gater, R., Campbell, M. and Jennett, N. (1996). The treatment of common mental disorders by a community team based in primary care: a cost-effectiveness study. *Psychological Medicine*, **26**, 487–92.

119 Eimerl, T.S. (1973). The E-book system for record keeping in general practice. *Medical Care*, **11**, 138–44.

120 Blythe, M. (2007). *Almost a Legend – John Fry*. London: Royal Society of Medicine.

121 Mackenzie, J. (1908). *Diseases of the Heart*. London: Henry Frowde, Hodder and Stoughton.

122 McMichael, J. (1981). Sir James MacKenzie and atrial fibrillation – a new perspective. *Journal of the Royal College of General Practitioners*, **31**, 402–6.

123 McCormick, J.S. (1981). Sir James MacKenzie and coronary heart disease. *Journal of the Royal College of General Practitioners*, **31**, 26–30.

124 Pickles, W. (1935). Epidemiology in Country Practice. *Proceedings of the Royal Society of Medicine*, **28**, 1337–42.

125 Pickles, W. (1936). Epidemic Catarrhal Jaundice with special reference to its epidemiology. *British Journal of Children's Diseases*, **33**, July–September.

126 Pemberton, J. ([1970] 1984). *Will Pickles of Wensleydale*. Geoffrey Bless, reprinted by the Royal College of General Practitioners.

127 Morrell, D.C., Gage, H.G. and Robinson, N.A. (1970). Patterns of demand in general practice. *Journal of the Royal College of General Practitioners*, **19**, 331–42.

128 Morrell, D.C. (1971). Experiences of morbidity in general practice. *British Medical Journal*, **2**, 454–8.

129 Morrell, D.C., Gage H.G. and Robinson N.A. (1971). Referral to hospital by general practitioners. *Journal of the Royal College of General Practitioners*, **21**, 77–85.

130 Morrell, D.C., Gage, H.G. and Robinson, N.A. (1971). Symptoms in general practice. *Journal of the Royal College of General Practitioners*, **21**, 32–43.

131 Morrell, D.C. (1970). Birth Update. *Journal of Postgraduate General Practice*, **2**, 931–2.

132 Morrell, D.C. and Kasap, H.S. (1972). The effect of an appointment system on demand for medical care. *International Journal of Epidemiology*, **1**, 143–51.

133 Zander, L.I., Beresford, A.A. and Thomas, P. (1978). *Medical Records in General Practice*. London: RCGP Occasional Paper No. 5.

134 Watkins, C.J. (1981). Medical audit in general practice: fact or fantasy. *Journal of the Royal College of General Practitioners*, **31**, 141–5.

135 Morrell, D.C. (1976). Symptoms perceived and recorded by patients. *Journal of the Royal College of General Practitioners*, **26**, 298–403.

136 Beresford, S.A.A., Waller, J.J., Banks, M.H. and Wale, C.J. (1977). Why do women consult doctors? Social factors and the use of general practitioners. *British Journal of Social and Preventive Medicine*, **31**, 220–226.

137 Banks, M.H. and Beresford, S.A.A. (1979). The influence of menstrual cycle phase upon symptoms recording using data from health diaries. *Journal of Psychosomatic Research*, 23, 307–13.

138 Zander, L.I. (1981). *Children's Illnesses*. Pocket Health Guides. London: Hamlyn Paperbacks.

139 Roland, M.O., Morrell, D.C. and Morris, R.W. (1983). Can general practitioners predict the outcome of back pain? *British Medical Journal*, **1**, 523–5.

140 Roland, M.O. and Morris, R.W. (1983). A study of the natural history of back pain. Part I. Development of a reliable and sensitive measure of disability in low back pain. Part 2. Development of guidelines for trials of treatment in primary care. *Spine*, **8**, 141–4 and 145–50.

141 Morrell, D.C., Avery, J.A. and Watkins, C.J. (1980). Management of minor illness. *British Medical Journal*, **280**, 769–71.

142 Sharp, D.S. (1992). *Childbirth Related Emotional Disorders in Primary Care. A Longitudinal Prospective Study.* PhD Thesis, University of London,.

143 Green, J. and Armstrong, D.A. (1993). Controlling the bed state: negotiating hospital organisation. *Sociology of Health and Illness*, **15**, 337–52.

144 Jenkins, C., Bartholomew, J., Gelder, F. and Morrell, D.C. (1994). Arranging hospital admission for acutely ill patients: problems encountered by general practitioners. *British Journal of General Practice*, **44**, 251–4.

145 Jankowski, R.F. and Mandalia, S. (1993). Comparison of attendance and emergency admission patterns of A&E departments in and out of London. *British Medical Journal*, **306**, 1241–3.

146 Britten, N. and Shaw, A. (1994). Patients' experiences of emergency admission: how relevant is the British Governments 'Patients Charter'? *Journal of Advanced Nursing*, **19**, 1212–20.

147 Savill, R. and Bartholomew, J. (1994). Planning better discharges. *Journal of Community Nursing*.

148 Byrne, P.S. (1975). Medical education and general practice. *Journal of the Royal College of General Practitioners*, **25**, 785–92.

149 Marinker, M. (1976). The family in medicine. *Proceedings of the Royal Society of Medicine*, **69**, 115–24.

150 Knox, J.D.E. (1976). Focus on learning in family practice. *Journal of the Royal College of General Practitioners*, **26**, 929–30.

151 Crombie, D.L. and Fleming D.M. (1986). Comparison of second national morbidity study and General Household Survey 1970–71. *Health Trends*, **18**, 15–18.

152 Pinsent, R.J.F.H. (1978). Continuous Morbidity Registration Sentinel Stations, Annual Report 1976. *Journal of the Royal College of General Practitioners*, **28**, 314–15.

153 Hope Simpson, R.E. (1981). Parainfluenza virus infections in the Cirencester Survey: seasonal and other characteristics. *Journal of Hygiene*, **87**, 393–406.

154 Josephs, L.K., Gregg, I. and Holgate, S.T. (1990). Does non-specific bronchial responsiveness indicate the severity of asthma. *European Respiratory Journal*, **3**, 220–227.

155 Kay, C.R. (1984). The Royal College of General Practitioners oral contraception study: some recent observations. *Clinics in Obstetrics and Gynaecology*, **11**, 759–86.

156 Medical Research Council Working Party (1985). MRC trial of treatment of mild hypertension: principal results. *British Medical Journal*, **291**, 97–104.

157 Holland, W.W. and Stewart, S. (1997). *Public Health. The Vision and the Challenge*. London: Nuffield Trust.

158 Topp, S.G., Cook, J., Holland, W.W. and Elliott, A. (1970). Influence of environmental factors on height and weight of schoolchildren. *British Journal of Preventive and Social Medicine*, **24**, 154–62.

159 Cook, J., Altman, D.G., Moore, D.M.C., Topp, S.G. and Holland, W.W. (1973). A nutritional survey of schoolchildren. *British Journal of Preventive and Social Medicine*, **27**, 91–9.

160 Rona, R.J. and Chinn, S. (1999). *The National Study of Health and Growth*. London: Oxford University Press.

161 Committee on Medical Aspects of Food Policy (1973). *Report by the Sub-Committee on Nutritional Surveillance*. London: Department of Health and Social Security.

162 Baker, I.A., Elwood, P.C., Hughes, J., Jones, M., Moore, F. and Sweetnam, P. (1980). A randomised controlled trial of the effect of the provision of free school milk on the growth of children. *Journal of Epidemiology and Community Health*, **34**, 31–4.

163 Peach, H., Green, S., Locker, D., Darby, S. and Patrick, D.L. (1980). Evaluation of a postal screening questionnaire to identify the physically disabled. *International Rehabilitation Medicine*, **2**, 189–93.

164 Patrick, D.L., Darby, S.C., Green, S., Horton, G., Locker, D. and Wiggins, R.D. (1981). Screening for disability in the inner city. *Journal of Epidemiology and Community Health*, **35**, 65–70.

165 Harris, A.I., Cox, E. and Smith, C.R.W. (1971). *National Survey of Disability. Part 1: Handicapped and Impaired in Great Britain. Part 2: Work and Housing of Impaired Persons in Great Britain*. Office of Population Censuses and Surveys. Social Survey Division. London: HMSO.

166 Charlton, J.R.H., Patrick, D.L. and Peach, H. (1983). Using multivariate measures of disability in community surveys. *Journal of Epidemiology and Community Health*, **37**, 296–304.

167 Sommerville, S.M., Silver, R. and Patrick, D.L. (1983). Services for disabled people. What criteria should we use to assess disability? *Community Medicine*, **5**, 302–10.

168 Morgan, M., Patrick, D.L. and Charlton, J. (1984). Social networks and psychosocial support among disabled people. *Social Science and Medicine*, **19**, 489–97.

169 Peach, H. (1984). Relationship between impairment and disability among disabled persons in the community. PhD thesis. University of London.

170 Patrick, D.L., Scrivens, E. and Charlton, J.R.H. (1983). Disability and patient satisfaction with medical care. *Medical Care*, **21**, 1062–75.

171 Locker, D. (1983). *Disability and Disadvantage: the Consequences of Chronic Illness*. London: Tavistock Publications.

172 Scrivens, E. and Caulfield, B. (1983). *Pilot study to Investigate Methods for Eliciting Consumer Preferences for Cash and Services*. Unpublished report to DHSS.

173 Great Britain, Ministry of Health, National Health Service (1962). A hospital plan for England and Wales. Cmnd 1604. London: HMSO.

174 Department of Health and Social Security (1976). *Sharing Resources for health in England. Report of the Resource Allocation Working Party.* London: HMSO.

175 DHSS (1970). Hospital Revenue Allocations. Paper RHB Chairmen 3/70. London: DHSS. Unpublished.

176 Mays, N. and Bevan, G. (1987). Resource Allocation in the Health Service. A review of the methods of the resource allocation working party (RAWP). Occasional Papers on Social Administration London: NCVO.

177 Bennett, A.E. and Holland, W.W. (1977). Rational planning or muddling through. *Lancet*, **1**, 464–6.

178 Palmer, S.R.R. (1978). The use of mortality data in resource allocation. In: Brotherston J. (ed.), *Morbidity and its Relationship to Resource Allocation: Papers and Proceeding of a Workshop held at Hill Residential College, Abergavenny, Gwent.* 24–25 January, pp. 25–39.

179 Holland, W.W. and Wainwright, A.H. (1979). Epidemiology and health policy. *Epidemiologic Reviews*, **1**, 211–32.

180 Palmer, S.R.R., West, P., Patrick, D. and Glynn, M. (1979). Mortality indices in resource allocation. *Community Medicine*, **1**, 275–81.

181 West, P.A. (1979). *Regional Equity in the National Health Service in England: an Economic Analysis of the Hospital Sector*. D.Phil. Thesis, University of York.

182 Palmer, S.R.R, West, P.A. and Dodd, P. (1980). Randomness in the RAWP formula: the reliability of mortality data in the allocation of NHS revenue. *Journal of Epidemiology and Community Health*, **34**, 212–16.

183 West, P.A., Palmer, S.R.R., Patrick, D. and Dodd, P. (1980). Sharing fairly in the NHS: the effects of imperfect cost data on RAWP. *Hospital and Health Services Review*, **76**, 330–334.

184 Carr Hill, R.A., Hardman, G., *et al.* (1994). *A Formula for Distributing NHS Revenues Based on Small Area Use of Hospital Beds*. York: York University Centre for Health Economics.

185 DHSS (1988). *Review of the Resource Allocation Working Party Formula. Final Report by the NHS Management Board*. London: HMSO.

186 Department of Health (1989). *Funding and Contracts for Health Services*. Working Paper No.2. London: HMSO.

187 Department of Health (1989). *Working for Patients. The Government's Review of the NHS.* London: HMSO.

188 Sheldon, T.A., Davey Smith, G. and Bevan, G. (1993). Weighting in the dark: resource allocation in the NHS. *British Medical Journal*, **306**, 835–9.

189 Mays, N. (1989). NHS resource allocation after the 1989 white paper. A critique of the research for the RAWP review. *Journal of Public Health*, **11**, 173–86.

190 Asthana, S., Gibson, A., Moon, G., Dicker, J. and Brigham, P. (2004). The pursuit of equity in NHS resource allocation: should morbidity replace utilisation as the basis for setting healthcare capitations? *Social Science and Medicine*, **58**, 539–51.

191 Department of Health (2008). *Report of the Advisory Committee on Resource Allocation.* Leeds: Department of Health.

192 Nuffield Trust (2009). *PBRA Report – Developing a Person-Based Resource Allocation Formula for Allocations to General Practices in England.* London: Nuffield Trust.

193 Glover, J.A. (1938). The incidence of tonsillectomy in schoolchildren. *Proceedings of the Royal Society of Medicine*, **31**, 1219–36.

194 Wennberg, J. and Gittelsohn, A. (1973). Small area variations in health care delivery. *Science*, **182**, 1102–8.

195 Donabedian, A. (1989). The end results of health care: Ernest Codman's contribution to quality assessment and beyond. *Milbank Memorial Fund Quarterly*, **67**(2), 233–56.

196 Lembcke, P.A. (1956). Medical auditing by scientific methods illustrated by major female pelvic surgery. *Journal of the American Medical Association*, **162**, 646–55.

197 Rutstein, D.D., Berenberg W., Chalmers, T.C., *et al.* (1976). Measuring the quality of medical care. *New England Journal of Medicine*, **294**, 582–8.

198 Rutstein, D.D., Berenberg, W., Chalmers, T.C., *et al.* (1980). Measuring the quality of medical care: second revision of tables of indexes. *New England Journal of Medicine*, **302**, 1146.

199 Charlton, J.R., Hartley, R.M., Silver, R. and Holland, W.W. (1983). Geographical variation in mortality from conditions amenable to medical intervention in England and Wales. *Lancet*, **1**, 691–6.

200 Osmon, T. (1983). Lottery of death. *The Sunday Times Magazine*, 18 September.

201 Holland, W.W. and Breeze, E. (1985). The performance of health services. In: Keynes, M., Coleman, D.A. and Dinsdale, N.H. (eds), *The Political Economy of Health and Welfare*. Proceedings of the 22nd Annual Symposium of the Eugenics Society. London: Macmillan Press, pp. 149–69.

202 MacFarlane, A. (2004). *Confidential Enquiries into Maternal Deaths: Development and Trends From 1952 Onwards.* 6th Report of Confidential Enquiries into Maternal Deaths in the UK. London: Royal College of Gynaecologists Press.

203 Godber, G. (1994). The origin and inception of the Confidential Enquiry into Maternal Deaths. *British Journal of Obstetrics and Gynaecology*, **101**, 946–7.

204   Holland, W.W. (2009). Measuring the quality of medical care. *Journal of Health Services Research* and *Policy*, **14**(3), 186–7.

205   Charlton, J.R., Holland, W.W., Lakhani, A. and Paul, E.A. (1987). Variations in avoidable mortality and variations in health care. *Lancet*, **1**, 858.

206   Holland, W.W. and Gardner, L. (1987). Measurement of outcome of district services. In: Greer, J. (ed.), *Quality and Performance. Proceedings of the Conference of the Faculty of Community Medicine 1986.* London: Faculty of Community Medicine (RCP) 2/4 1–7.

207   Holland, W.W. (1990). Avoidable death as a measure of quality. *Quality Assurance Health Care*, **2**, 227–33.

208   Holland, W.W. (ed.) (1988). *European Community Atlas of Avoidable Death.* London: Oxford University Press.

209   Holland, W.W. (ed.) (1991). *European Community Atlas of Avoidable Death.* Second Edition, Volume I. Oxford: Oxford Medical Publications.

210   Holland, W.W. (ed.) (1993). *European Community Atlas of Avoidable Death.* Second Edition, Volume II. Oxford: Oxford Medical Publications.

211   Charlton, J.R.H., Bauer, R. and Lakhani, A.R. (1984). Outcome measures for district and regional health care planners. *Journal of Public Health Medicine*, **6**, 306–15.

212   Charlton, J.R.G. and Velez, R. (1986). Some international comparisons of mortality amenable to medical intervention. *British Medical Journal*, **292**, 295–301.

213   Nolte, E. and McKee, M. (2004). *Does Health Care Save Lives? Avoidable Mortality Revisited.* London: Nuffield Trust.

7. Priorities in medical research: the House of Lords Select Committee

INTRODUCTION

Concern with the funding of medical research came very much to the fore in the mid-1980s. Medical researchers expressed their anxieties both about the money available as well as about the organisation and management of research. This was the era of a Conservative administration under Margaret Thatcher. The government was very much concerned with public expenditure which they maintained had increased considerably under Callaghan and Wilson in the 1970s. The NHS and medical research were easy targets for reduction of expenditure and, although there was no actual reduction in the money spent on these areas, the rate of increase was reduced. This meant that there was a perceived dearth of funds, as described in Chapter 5, and there was a great deal of unrest, particularly in the medical profession.

A number of questions and debates in the Houses of Parliament resulted in the House of Lords Select Committee on Science and Technology forming a subcommittee on *Priorities in Medical Research*.[1-3]

The Committee was chaired by Lord Nelson of Stafford, Chairman of the large electrical company GEC, and had 13 other members (see Table 7.1). Six of these had a health background – nursing, physiology, general practice, medicine and pharmacology – one was an ethicist, one a chemist and one a noted mathematician and computer expert. Three had experience of university administration as Vice-Chancellors. The rest were drawn from other backgrounds and included a former head of the Foreign Office. There were two specialist advisers – Sir John Butterfield, former Regius Professor of Physic at the University of Cambridge, and myself. The Committee was administered by a Clerk of the House of Lords with appropriate secretarial help.

Table 7.1   Members of the House of Lords Subcommittee

Member's Name	Expertise
Lord Adrian	Physiology
Lord Erroll of Hale	Engineering and Politics
Lord Flowers	Mathematics, Computing, University Administration
Lord Hunter of Newington	Materia Medica, University Administration
Lord Kearton	Chemistry, Industry
Baroness Lockwood	Education, Politics
Baroness McFarlane of Llandaff	Nursing
Lord Nelson of Stafford (Chairman)	Industry
Lord Perry of Walton	Pharmacology, University Administration
Lord Rea	General Practice
Lord Sherfield	Civil Service
Lord Smith	Surgery
Lord Taylor of Blackburn	Education, Law, Local Politics
Baroness Warnock	Ethics
Specialist Advisers	
Sir John Butterfield	Medicine, University Administration
Professor Walter W. Holland	Public Health Medicine

The Committee visited two London Medical Schools (University College and Middlesex Hospital Medical School and United Medical and Dental School of Guy's and St Thomas' Hospitals), the Royal College of Physicians of Edinburgh, the Trent Regional Health Authority, Sheffield, and the Imperial Cancer Research Fund Laboratories in Lincoln's Inn Fields, London. In addition, four members of the Committee and one specialist adviser visited eight universities in the US as well as the US National Institutes of Health, the US Department of Health and Human Services, the US Institute of Medicine, the US Office of Management and Budget, and the Rand Corporation.

Evidence was requested from all UK universities, medical charities, Royal Colleges and their Faculties, Health Authorities, as well as a large number of individuals. Written evidence was received from more than 200 individuals and institutions and 42 of these also gave oral evidence.

The written evidence was reviewed by all members of the Committee, including the specialist advisers, and the oral witnesses were largely chosen on the basis of the replies they had submitted (see Volumes 2 and 3 of the Report[2, 3]). In addition, the Medical Research Council, the Economic and Social Research Council (ESRC) and the Department of Health, including Ministers, were interviewed.

The specialist advisers did not take part in the oral interviews. Their role was to advise the Chairman and Committee members on what questions to ask and plan the oral meetings, but also to pass written suggestions and supplementary questions to the Committee to probe further or follow-up on the answers provided.

As one of the specialist advisers I was immensely impressed by the intelligence and expertise of all members of the Committee. The shrewdness of their judgements, both on individuals and evidence presented, was remarkable. The comments on individuals who presented their views to the specialist advisers cannot be divulged as they were confidential, but the ability to identify the knowledge and intelligence of the witnesses as well as their gaps in logic was uncanny, and often far more to the point than that of the specialist advisers – who were supposed to be the experts in the field!

Much of what follows is in the form of direct quotation from Volume 1 of the Report.[1]

The conclusions of the Committee were radical. The major finding was that there was a collapse in the morale of researchers because of the obstacles to research created by the Department of Health as well as the NHS:

> the impression, right or wrong, is that neither the DHSS nor the NHS demonstrates any awareness of the importance of research nor is prepared to devote time, effort and resources to promote it, save only when either an immediate saving of money is in prospect or when public concern, as in the case of Aids, forces its hand (para 3.1). (HL Papers 54-I)[1]

The Report continued:

> in priorities for medical research two crucial if negative truths stand out. First, priorities do not announce themselves, either in theory or in practice; and secondly, it is by no means obvious what the needs of the National Health Service are (para 3.3).
>
> Although, on the face of it, ministerial policy might define the needs of the NHS for the purpose of setting research priorities, it cannot in fact do so. The

Johnson and Nixon initiatives against heart disease and cancer in the United States show that government action, on however generous a scale, is not all that is needed to solve health problems. Throwing money at a problem in the absence of promising ideas will not bring about any breakthrough. Nor can intervention at the national level identify the more detailed service needs of the NHS. Indeed, without criticism of either party, the Committee draw a clear distinction between ministerial policy and NHS research needs. They are not necessarily the same. Medical research has to inform departmental policy as much as be directed by it (para 3.4).

Better health for all is the goal, but it is not a clear one. The evidence put to the Committee reveals real differences of approach as to how better health is to be achieved, or even about what it consists of. Should medical research concentrate on cure or prevention? Which approach will in the long term yield greater benefits? How are benefits to be measured for the purpose of establishing priorities? These questions have complex answers. Because of that complexity, any formal mechanism for directing national priorities would almost certainly be inefficient and could stifle research. Instead the Committee prefer to rely on pluralistic funding and administration of research, in which good ideas compete for support. The aggregate of decisions taken by different interests is more likely to reflect the balance of needs and opportunities in research than a centrally directed research effort, provided that the different interests are aware of each other's priorities (para 3.5).

The Committee also consider that medical research and medical education should be inseparable. They recommend that medical research should continue to be carried out for the most part in, or in association with, the medical schools and universities, rather than in national centres. There are four reasons for this. First, research cannot easily be separated from hospitals because of the demands of clinical research. Secondly, the growing interdisciplinary and inter-faculty nature of medical research, and its dependence on a critical mass of different disciplines, makes a broad academic base desirable. Thirdly, the bulk of research funded by the medical charities, and indeed industry, should as far as possible be carried out in the same places as MRC-funded research, so that they are not isolated from one another. Fourthly, medical research and education should continue to stimulate each other (para 3.7).

The Committee reject, in the specific case of medical research, the Association of British Research Councils' (ABRC) proposal for the ranking of higher education institutions because this would imply that some medical schools could be run on a teaching-only basis (para 3.8). (HL Papers 54-I)[1]

SCIENCE-LED OR PROBLEM-LED MEDICAL RESEARCH?

Rothschild's 1970s argument about the need for research to be carried out to answer specific questions was also tackled:

Implicit in much of the evidence received by the Committee are two different approaches to medical research. One is science-led: it emphasises the role of the individual researcher (or research team) in developing new lines of enquiry. The other is problem-led: it emphasises the need to study the current health status of the population, and present methods of treatment, as a means both of directing research towards the problems with the most serious effects, and of ensuring that medical practice, whether existing or new, is the best possible (para 3.9).

In other areas of civil science the recent trend has been towards problem-led research, with emphasis on strategic targets for research and focussing on specific applications or practical opportunities, while preserving a sound level of basic research, The Committee have endorsed this trend most recently in their report on Civil Research and Development (para 3.10).

But the accepted wisdom of biomedical research is that the science-led approach should be dominant. The Committee take the same view. Better results will be achieved by supporting good ideas and advances in science as they arise, than by concentrating on recognised problems regardless of whether promising leads are in prospect. More than one witness (para 2.2) drew attention to the work of Comroe and Dripps and their demonstration of the importance of maintaining a high level of science-led basic biomedical research on the grounds of the historical significance of serendipity in medical science (para 3.11).

The Committee therefore recommend that the main focus of public policy in medical research should be the establishment of a strong infrastructure for research in well-found laboratories and the supply of a strongly motivated and well trained research community. This, in theory at least, is the existing system. When new problems are identified and priorities change, research leaders should be encouraged to move to the new areas in order to build up scientific strength and the new research teams. But the tradition of investigator initiated medical research should be preserved (para 3.12).

On the other hand a wholly science-led approach cannot be effective. Some decisions about priorities have to be taken, particularly when good scientific ideas outnumber the funds available to pursue them. The NHS has changing needs and priorities must reflect this. The public rightly expects a response to new problems such as AIDS. A system which relies on the initiative of individual scientists will develop gaps and those can become self-perpetuating: funds go to the best people and the best people are then attracted to well-funded areas. Potential gaps have to be identified early if research teams are to be built up in the right specialities (para 3.13). (HL Papers 54-I)[1]

The need for a multiplicity of sources for research funding with the concomitant need to coordinate was addressed:

As the funding of medical research has come to rely on several sources (indicated in paragraph 1.10) and is not dominated by any of them, so the need to make each aware of the interests of the others is becoming more apparent. The MRC, for instance, needs to know where work is being planned by the charities; both have to be aware of the requirements of the NHS; all stand to gain from a knowledge of what research is going on in industry; and the Health Departments must be conscious of the overall shape of research effort and the gaps which may be developing. The DES and the Health Departments ought to be acutely aware of the interactive effect of their respective policies on medical education, training and research (para 3.14).

This suggests that some setting of priorities and some emphasis on problem-led research is essential. The Committee believe so. Yet remarkably there appears to be no coherent means of setting priorities beyond that which is provided by the MRC in discussions with the DHSS. This is becoming gradually less effective as these bodies account for a shrinking proportion of national spending on medical research. The lead from the DHSS is weak, in contrast with the approach of the Scottish Home and Health Department. The only body which appears to accept some responsibility for supporting underfunded areas of research is the Wellcome Trust. The Committee do not believe that Governments should rely on charities to fill gaps in national research effort. The remedies proposed by the Committee are described in chapter 4 (para 3.15). (HL Papers 54-I)[1]

APPLIED RESEARCH

The Committee's reservations about existing priorities in medical research in the United Kingdom begin where the MRC's responsibility for basic research shades into its responsibility for clinical research. The Committee have received some evidence which suggests that the MRC is not as vigorous in pursuing the latter as it is in pursuing basic research; the MRC denied this (paras 2.28–30). The Committee noted that the Clinical Research Centre (CRC) at Northwick Park has represented a major commitment by the MRC to clinical research: they assume that this commitment will continue after whatever institutional changes that are planned for the CRC have been effected. The Committee were moreover convinced, especially following their visit to America, that there is no real conceptual divide between basic and academic clinical research. The Committee however feel that, since clinical research involves patients and patient care, this begins to move away from the basic science field which belongs to the Research Councils and different considerations apply. These considerations are bound up with the administration of clinical research, and the special demands it makes: the patients are cared for, often under regimes which are more complex and expensive than normal regimes of care; and that a significant number of the researchers involved must be clinicians (para 3.16).

The Committee consider that the main defects of the present system lie in applied research and in the application of knowledge gained from research. Therefore they begin by recommending that the MRC should take pains to strengthen the contribution of clinicians to its work. The Committee, in what follows, have no wish to disturb the responsibilities of the MRC or its funding, nor to create an artificial division in the continuum of basic and clinical research supported by the MRC. But the MRC must spend effectively those funds returned to it under the 'concordat' in 1981 and counter any tendency to concentrate too much on basic research when funds are short. As new techniques, particularly in molecular biology, pervade the whole range of medical research and become standard diagnostic tools, the MRC's awareness of the clinical applications of basic research should be emphasised (para 3.17). (HL Papers 54-I)[1]

NHS

The funding of applied research in medicine is known to be troublesome. This was demonstrated by the abortive transfer of funds from the MRC to the DHSS following the Rothschild Report and their subsequent return to the MRC. But the situation is still unsatisfactory. In the Committee's opinion, the key lies not in the DHSS but in the NHS (para 3.18).

The NHS is inextricably involved with medical research. It is responsible for the health of the nation in which research has a vital role. It is the ultimate customer for nearly all medical research, whether funded by the MRC, the charities, the pharmaceutical and medical equipment industries or done in the NHS itself. Practically all clinical research is carried out in NHS hospitals; it involves clinicians on NHS contracts (whether they are NHS clinicians or academics on honorary contracts), NHS nursing and ancillary staff, and NHS patients. Teaching hospitals provide the tertiary referral facilities for many parts of the country because of their academic and clinical strength in various specialities. The NHS has to absorb the consequences of successful research: better health care may often involve more expensive treatment, though not necessarily; research will sometimes produce cheaper treatment. Last, but by no means least, the resources on which clinical medical and dental education are based are the NHS's responsibility (para 3.19).

Yet medical research and the health services have come to be administered separately. There are good historical and theoretical reasons why medical education and research take place in universities and are the responsibility eventually of the DES. But administrative remoteness of medical research from the NHS is a source of weakness to both sides (para 3.20).

In particular there has been a serious divergence of administrative approaches between medical research and medical services in the United Kingdom. Medical research requires critical masses of expertise and expensive equipment in particular locations, normally with access to large centres of population. By contrast NHS policy has been to disperse such unequal centres of excellence (which provide the privilege of exceptional service to those with access to them) in favour of providing a service of equal standard throughout the United Kingdom. The effect of this policy, pursued through the Resource Allocation Working Party (RAWP) process, has been to harm some centres of medical research excellence. Through RAWP the NHS funds which used to be concentrated in the great London and provincial teaching hospitals have been more evenly distributed throughout the country. Within Regional Health Authorities teaching districts have also lost their privileged budgets to some degree. While this shift in resources has brought about service benefits and some expansion of research in some provincial centres, the overall effect on medical research, which depends on concentrated excellence, has been a contraction, particularly in the London hospitals; and this has been compounded by cutbacks in general University Grants Committee (UGC) funding. The two dual funding systems (para 1.10) have thus been working against one another (para 3.21).

The Committee believe that no research system can function effectively when the principal customer for research has so small a direct input into the initiation of research programmes. First, neither the NHS nor the DHSS spends much, in comparative terms, on research. The main funding bodies are the MRC, charities and industry, each with an orientation different from that of the NHS. Secondly, as long as medical research is primarily initiated by the researchers, the needs of the NHS and its problems will be met only if those needs are clearly expressed. The needs are not so expressed (para 3.22).

The Committee recognise that many administrative links exist between medical research and the DHSS. In particular, since the 'concordat' of 1981, there has been an annual 'stocktaking' meeting, an account of which is published in the annual DHSS Handbook of Research and Development. Representatives of the MRC and all the Health Departments attend this meeting. The Office of the Chief Scientist in the DHSS and the Scottish Office provide other links, and this can be a successful mechanism, where the scale is right, as in the Scottish Home and Health Department (para 3.23).

The DHSS is however not to be identified with the administration of the NHS, in spite of the intimacy of their relationship. The Committee were dismayed by the description of the purpose of the DHSS research programme given by the Chief Scientist: 'The main aim of DHSS health research is to provide guidance to Ministers on ways of improving the efficiency and effectiveness of the health and personal social services by promoting improvements in organisation, operation and administration.'(p. 410 [Volume 2]). Ministers need a research programme, obviously. The NHS needs a research programme also, and it is likely to be different, both in scale and kind (para 3.24).

The Committee do not underestimate the NHS's local interest in research. NHS managers, whether at Regional or District level, have freedom to commission the research they need from their own allocations; the Regional Health Authorities have notional research budgets within their overall allocations; and Regions have Research Committees which administer the Locally Organised Research Scheme. The Committee applaud the arrangements described to them during their visit to the Trent RHA, which has been a relative gainer from the RAWP process over the last few years. The RHA has given extra support to research with these funds. Within the Region there are three medical schools, two of them – those at Nottingham and Leicester – only a few years old. In Sheffield alone there is a medical school, a joint MRC/ESRC Research Unit, and a DHSS/RHA Unit. A good illustration of the sensitivity of the Trent RHA to the needs of academic medicine has been a regional readjustment of the SIFT allocation to the teaching districts to take account of the demands on them (para 3.25).

However, without entering the public dispute about funding of the NHS as a whole, the Committee see that those working in the NHS are increasingly hard pressed to maintain a level of service and this directly affects research. Clinicians are being diverted from research by the demands of patient care while medical staff and management alike have less opportunity to understand, disseminate and implement research results. Symptomatic of the NHS's lack of awareness of research needs are the following: the first report of the Hayhoe Committee made no provision for the honorary NHS contracts needed by medical researchers; there appear to be no administrative efforts on the part of the NHS to prevent service pressures from constantly eroding the research time of clinician researchers; no formal consideration is given to the level of spending on medical research compared with the level of service spending; the new White Paper on primary health care contains no proposals for a rigorous research programme either to develop primary care further or to access the wider effects of the changes now being introduced (para 3.26).

Too much is left to chance in ensuring firstly that the NHS plays its part in formulating its research needs and supporting medical researchers in meeting those needs and secondly that the NHS is aware of what research is being done in the UK (para 3.27).

The Committee's central recommendation is that the NHS should be brought into the mainstream of medical research. The NHS should articulate its research needs; it should assist in meeting those needs; and it should ensure that the fruits of research are systematically transferred into service (para 4.1).

Up to a point the Committee have identified the same failing that Lord Rothschild's report sought to correct in enunciating the customer/contractor principle. The NHS is the main customer for research results and so it should commission research for which it perceives a need. But this oversimplified proposition has to be qualified: The distinction between basic and applied research is blurred, and the initiative in the best biomedical research is likely to arise among the scientists rather than the service administrators. The NHS, both as customer and as the provider of hospital facilities and patients, has to complement the work of the MRC and other funding bodies, not to displace them. Therefore the Committee's proposal outlined below differs in two vital respects from that put into effect by the Government in 1971, after the Rothschild Report. It does not involve withdrawing money from the MRC; and it places the primary responsibility for applied research with the NHS, not the Health Departments (para 4.2).

The Committee consider this to be an opportune time to recommend an adjustment to the organisation of the NHS since the matter is actively under consideration in government. The development of NHS management with its own Board and with functional authorities for Health Education and Training (for management) highlights the absence of any identified research function in the NHS. An opportunity to improve the efficiency and cost-effectiveness of the service is being missed. The Chief Scientist's Office in DHSS may be adequate for the Department's internal purposes but it has certainly not proved

capable of supplying the informed customer for health research envisaged by
Lord Rothschild (para 4.3).

In order to meet the objectives of para 4.1 above, and on the grounds of
efficiency and cost-effectiveness, the Committee recommend the creation of a
new special health authority within the NHS, to which they refer hereafter as
the National Health Research Authority (NHRA) (para 4.4). (HL Papers
S4-I)[1]

NATIONAL HEALTH RESEARCH AUTHORITY (NHRA)

The Committee stress that the NHRA should form an integral part of the NHS
structure, as a special health authority equivalent to the RHAs. It should be
organisationally – and physically – separated from the DHSS. The new Health
Education Authority (HEA) and the National Health Service Training Authority (NHSTA) provide some organisational models for special authorities
undertaking distinct functions for the NHS as a whole. If the structure of the
NHS were radically altered, there would remain a need for a central agency to
carry out the functions which the Committee propose for the NHRA. There
should be arrangements for the functions of the NHRA to be carried out
throughout the United Kingdom. These arrangements would obviously provide for close liaison between the NHRA and any equivalent body carrying
out its functions in Scotland, Wales and Northern Ireland (para 4.5). (HL
Papers 54-I)[1]

PUBLIC HEALTH AND OPERATIONAL RESEARCH

The Committee used the term Public Health and Operational Research
rather than simply HSR because of possible ambiguities. But their
recommendations for this form of research were very clear.

The Committee consider that public health research and operational research
have been inadequately supported in the United Kingdom. It is especially
serious that so large an organisation as the NHS devotes so small a part of its
budget to seeking how to improve its own operations. To secure a research
capability in public health and operational research, the Committee recommend that the NHRA should foster at least three centres for these disciplines,
ideally linked to medical schools in different parts of the country. This would
involve an expansion and consolidation of the units already funded by the
DHSS and the Scottish Home and Health Department (para 4.12).

The Committee believe that this would encourage the long-term development of public health and operational research, by providing a flow of
research contracts and career prospects capable of drawing talented researchers into the subject. The Committee have no doubt that these are areas of
research which would repay – literally repay – investment. The Committee

recommend that spending in these areas should therefore be markedly increased. What they propose would also supply the NHS with a number of institutions capable of producing first-class independent academic work which is attuned to the needs of the Health Service and the Health Departments. Another important advantage the Committee foresee arising out of these centres is that they would provide a pool of able people with experience and knowledge of the working of the NHS from among whom future NHS managers can be recruited (para 4.13).

The Committee believe that these recommendations underpin, rather than duplicate, the recommendations made in the Acheson Report on Public Health in England. In particular the recommendations in the Acheson Report for a small unit to be established within the DHSS bringing together relevant disciplines and skills to monitor the health of the public will not be replicated by the NHRA. The latter's research base would help the DHSS unit to fulfil its 'primary object ... to provide more effective support to the Secretary of State.' Monitoring of health is not enough: systematic public health research has to be undertaken. The Committee regret the limited extent of the recommendations on public health research in the Acheson Report (para 4.14).

Particularly in relation to public health research, the Committee stress the importance of the right to publish in maintaining academic independence and the standards of research. They were not entirely reassured by the Minister of Health's statement about the revision of DHSS research contracts in the light of Crown copyright (Q 2190). The DHSS and the NHRA should safeguard the right of academics to publish research commissioned from them, subject only to legitimate delay in order to safeguard intellectual property rights (para 4.15). (HL Papers 54-I)[1]

USE OF COMMERCIAL CONSULTANTS BY THE NHS

Another problem which several groups had mentioned was the use by the NHS of external, commercial consultants or management consultants.

Since the NHRA would be the principal means of developing the first-class management and operational research base which the NHS needs, the Committee believe that the NHRA should be the channel through which the NHS commissions research centrally from management consultants. In some cases it may be that properly managed academic contracts could be better value for money than contracts with commercial consultants. The use of commercial consultants should not be pursued as a short-term expedient in such a way as to restrict the growth of specialised centres of operational research expertise. It is moreover essential that, where commercial consultants are used, it is on the same basis, with the same research management, assessment and review, as other sources of research (para 4.16). (HL Papers 54-I)[1]

FUNDING OF THE NHRA

The question of funding was also tackled and the Committee members on several occasions expressed their surprise at how little was spent compared to the amount spent by industry on research to maintain its competitiveness. They considered that the amount spent on research in relation to the costs of the NHS was far too small – and suggested a minimum of about 1.5 per cent of the running costs of the NHS.

> The Committee believe that the funding for the NHRA should come from the DHSS Vote. The activities of the NHRA should not diminish the area of responsibility of the MRC enough to justify the return of the Rothschild funds (or any portion of them) to the DHSS for the purpose of funding the NHRA. Such a transfer should be contemplated only if failure by the MRC to fund clinical research led to a great increase in the funding of academic clinical research by the NHRA (para 4.22).
>
> The Committee recommend that the NHRA take over the bulk of the budget of £8 million at present spent by the DHSS on health services research. The Office of the Chief Scientist would keep that element of its budget needed for research in support of ministerial policy, rather than NHS research. The NHRA would take on the management of most of the health service units and projects at present in that programme (para 4.23).
>
> The NHRA's responsibility for the administration of NHS research would involve it taking over certain administrative tasks from other DHSS and NHS institutions. This should be recognised in the NHRA's resource allocation (para 4.24).
>
> In addition the Committee believe that the NHRA should in part be funded out of Regional allocations. They envisage something along the lines of a subscription from RHAs to the NHRA. Regional Health Authorities would make a mandatory contribution, to be set by the Secretary of State, but should be free to finance the NHRA to a greater extent if they desire, and to attach specific conditions to such a funding if they wish. The Committee recommend this system as a means of introducing an element of accountability into the NHRA's funding and of associating the NHRA closely with the RHAs. The NHRA will be successful in so far as it proves useful to RHAs (para 4.25). (HL Papers 54-I)[1]

The Committee looked at a number of other areas such as relations with (and support by) the Medical Charities, the need for research in the medical and equipment industries, as well as the role, and its research, of nurses and other non-medical personnel. They tackled the question of manpower and identified a need for proper training facilities as well as a career structure for HSR researchers. One of their recommendations was that more money should be given to develop "programmes" of research and encourage coherent projects to improve health care rather than to support individual project grants. This would enable a more stable environment to be created for researchers as well as increasing their productivity as they did not continuously have to look for support.

REACTION TO THE REPORT

The Report of this Enquiry was well received by the academic research community. Unfortunately the central recommendation of the Committee to create a National Health Research Authority funded by the NHS, for which the research is carried out, was not accepted by the Government.[4] Instead it proposed the appointment of a Chief of R&D who was to advise and act for the Secretary of State for Health across the whole range of research interests. The Chief of R&D was to hold a senior post and to take on the task of advising the NHS Management Executive on priorities for NHS research and managing this, and to create a NHS regional structure for identifying and meeting clinical and service research needs.

Obviously the Lords' Committee was unhappy with this response since it would perpetuate the inability of the NHS to identify and support relevant research and the dominance of the political rather than service need for research.

With some effective persuasion the Government was at least persuaded that a Director of R&D should be appointed, with Second Permanent Secretary status, commensurate with the responsibility for research. The Director of R&D was, in addition, to be a member, not only an adviser, of the NHS Management Executive. This was some advance on the Government's initial response, but did not really achieve the far-seeing vision of the House of Lords.

The Lords' Committee had recognised the great need for HSR to be used by the NHS. It felt that the only way to do this would be for the NHS to have a body responsible for such research, and to pay for it – and thus use it. The need to remove HSR from the dead hand of political control was considered, on past experience over the last ten years, to be beneficial, in contrast to the first years between 1968 and 1973 when there was interest and sympathy for such research, with the backing of Sir George Godber, the Chief Medical Officer of the time.

The new structure of a Director of R&D as a member of the NHS Management Board was an improvement. But individuals not responsible for the delivery of services were still in control. This meant that the NHS was still not closely involved in either the identification or commissioning of research needs, in spite of the creation of a number of committees charged with this task. The Director of R&D also appointed a number of individuals as Regional Directors of Research – most were medical academics, with one (out of 14) a Professor of Social Medicine. Their task was to facilitate research and to identify areas for this. The problem of freedom to publish was tackled with the use of copyright law and intellectual property. However the need to tackle the problems of training, manpower, career security and appropriate mix of disciplines involved remained unresolved.

The thinking underlying the new arrangements is described by Peckham, the first Director of R&D, in his Rock Carling Lecture of 2000.[5] One of the major tasks undertaken by the Director of R&D was to compile a catalogue of current and past HSR and the Cochrane Centre was also established in Oxford to assess the validity of evidence on which decisions on the practice of medicine could be based.

Over the years there have been many further developments and reorganisations of research and these are beyond the scope of this book. Events since the Report appeared illustrate how much good HSR continues to be needed. Recent changes in 2009–2010 in the methods of health care delivery through the Darzi centres (see Postscript), introduction of unevaluated health screening measures for diabetes and cardiovascular disease and the increasing use of management consultants to undertake unevaluated work are all testament to this need. There is little doubt that, in diluting the recommendations of the Lords Select Committee, the Government of the day missed a real opportunity to lay a sound and sustainable foundation for the future of HSR in the UK.

REFERENCES

1 House of Lords Select Committee on Science and Technology (1988). *Priorities in Medical Research: Volume 1 Report.* London: HMSO.
2 House of Lords Select Committee on Science and Technology (1988). *Priorities in Medical Research: Volume 2 Oral Evidence.* London: HMSO.
3 House of Lords Select Committee on Science and Technology (1988). *Priorities in Medical Research: Volume 3 Written Evidence.* London: HMSO.
4 Department of Health (1989). *Priorities in Medical Research. Government Response to the Third Report of the House of Lords Select Committee on Science and Technology: 1987–88 Session.* London: HMSO.
5 Peckham M. (2000). *A Model for Health Innovation and the Future of Health Services.* London: Nuffield Provincial Hospitals Trust.

8. Key questions

INTRODUCTION

Many difficulties arise in the conduct of HSR. One fundamental problem is how to ensure that those involved in commissioning such research and implementing its findings fully understand its nature – what it can and cannot do. Researchers in this field are equipped to tackle precise rather than general questions.

On the matter of manpower substitution, for example, those involved in policy formulation might want to know whether nurses could be used instead of doctors in the primary care setting. This question is far too vague and general to form a productive avenue for research. A nurse would be well equipped to deal with some primary care contacts, such as minor injury or simple triage of abdominal pain in a child. But that nurse might not be able to decide whether the abdominal pain required laparotomy or was indicative of acute appendicitis.

So the research question must be specific – can nurses rather than doctors be used to handle patients with respiratory tract problems or with abrasions, and what back-up is required for them to be able to identify, for example, a serious fracture underlying an abrasion?

Since the number of questions asked is infinite, it is crucial that the researcher is involved in determining the objective of a piece of research. The policy-maker must also accept that, in order to answer a particular question, it may be necessary to synthesise from the research findings and to investigate a few specific examples to illuminate the problem, rather than to provide a definitive solution.

An illustration of this can be seen in the question that the St Thomas' Unit was asked about whether the 'best-buy' hospital design of changing the emphasis from inpatient to outpatient care would be satisfactory. This was such a wide-ranging remit that to provide a meaningful answer we had to attempt to disentangle certain components of change from inpatient to outpatient care.

Shortening length of stay after surgery would, inevitably, decrease the inpatient facilities required, as long as the void was not filled by further work or operations (see Chapter 6). Local surgeons were willing to carry out a randomised controlled trial of short-stay (one to two days) after hernia or varicose vein operations compared with normal practice which, at that time, was a stay of at least seven days in hospital. This trial demonstrated that patients did not mind being discharged early, that there was no increase in complications or side effects, but that, although NHS costs were reduced, the total 'social cost' which included the cost to families as well as social security for time off work, did not differ greatly between the two groups. This was largely because the major 'social' cost was the payments to the patient for time off work and this did not differ between the two groups. One further consequence of early discharge was that nurses' work increased – partly because the number of patients in a convalescent stage and thus needing less attention diminished – and because of the early discharge there was a greater intensity of work required to cope with the patients in the early stages of recovery who needed help. Furthermore, with early discharge fewer patients were available to help with chores on the ward, such as handing round cups of tea and distributing mail or newspapers. Thus we were able to recommend that the 'best-buy' model of care, by reducing surgical post-operative stay, was acceptable to patients and did not lead to an increase in complications but did result in an increased workload for hospital staff. Although this study was confined to an examination of a change of policy in two relatively minor operations, it was likely that the results would also apply to other minor surgical procedures. We had chosen hernia and varicose vein operations because they represented a significant burden on the surgical caseload and there were enough operations to enable a randomised controlled trial to be carried out over a short time period.

For medical conditions we chose quite different problems to illuminate the change in practice. Stroke is a relatively common occurrence, particularly in the elderly. At the time of our study it was a much neglected condition. Most patients with a stroke were warehoused into hospital and received little, if any, treatment or rehabilitation. Because of the neglect of this condition, few figures were available of incidence, resource needs after onset of an episode or long-term consequences. With the help of all the local general practitioners, we established a system in which any patient who developed the symptoms of a stroke in their practice was identified, recorded and followed for two to three years. We were thus able to establish the incidence of different severities of stroke, their natural history and resource needs. We showed that about one-third of stroke patients died within one month. Of those who survived a large proportion recovered to the extent that their functional ability was the same as before their stroke. This provided the local health care managers with a true estimate of the need for inpatient facilities for individuals with a severe chronic disability illness and showed how much rehabilitation services could do to enable patients to return to their previous state at home.

The general practitioners around the Frimley area, where the new hospital was sited, had used four small community hospitals for their patients who required inpatient care. Admitting privileges were to be continued in the new hospital as the community hospitals would close, but it was not known what type of patients were being admitted under their own GP and what ancillary facilities, including X-ray and laboratory investigations, were needed for these patients. To explore this we carried out an observational study in which the diagnoses and resource requirements of patients admitted under the care of a GP were compared with those admitted under a consultant. It was shown, as expected, that, in general, the patients in consultant care had more complex diagnoses than those in GP care. For many of the patients with similar diagnoses, such as pneumonia or heart failure, however, for those admitted under GP care far fewer X-ray or laboratory tests were requested than for those admitted under a consultant. This study was thus able to provide guidance about the number of GP care beds needed, as well as the resources required to meet their investigational needs.

The series of studies in relation to 'best-buy' options was able to provide general guidance of resource requirements and what the consequences of changes in practice would be. It should be noted that the researchers chose specific problems with definable end points in relation to the very general question of the consequences of change of emphasis from inpatient to community care. It should also be emphasised that local practitioners were involved in both the design and execution of the studies so that they 'owned' them, accepted the findings and were willing to change their practice. The amount of effort required by the researchers to involve local personnel of all grades should not be underestimated. We were fortunate that several of the opinion leaders in the area came from our medical school and thus trusted us not impose unnecessary changes. This lesson of involving local personnel in altering accepted practice is crucial if change is to occur. It is unfortunate that this is currently often neglected, leading to great difficulties in the implementation of change.

IMPORTANCE OF COORDINATION

The enormous range of problems that HSR needs to tackle means that it is unlikely that it can provide answers to more than a small proportion and it is essential to consider how best to use the scarce available research resources. As described above, the Rothschild proposals of distinguishing between pure or basic research and the more applied research were promulgated in 1971. Many politicians and administrators felt that the arrangements under which almost all health research was funded by the Medical Research Council was inadequate because that body was mainly concerned with basic research, considered more prestigious than research concerned with mundane problems of organisation or of an applied nature. I have already described the tortuous development of research funding since the end of the First World War. But recognition of the need for pragmatic solutions to enable research to serve society in a useful way had been neglected. In the St Thomas' Unit we were able to develop a successful model which enabled researchers, administrators, policy-makers and practitioners to work together amicably and productively. This, of course did not work on all occasions. The best example of its failure was in the evaluation of lithotripsy where the surgeons, after initial agreement, refused to undertake a randomised controlled trial (see Chapter 6).

HSR results can be applied either at a local level, to influence change in practice or organisation in a practice, hospital or authority, or at a central level to influence or evaluate general policy – for example, advice on health hazards such as smoking, or on the organisation and delivery of health services.

We were engaged in research at both levels. As described in Chapter 6, one research project of health care in Lambeth was designed to illuminate the resources needed to satisfy the needs of the local population. We rapidly discovered that it was essential to develop links to the local health administration (at that time there was a Hospital Board of Governors and a Local Health Authority). The Board of Governors also identified that there might be advantages in developing formal links between the Research Unit and the Hospital Administration. The Clerk of Governors (the chief hospital executive's title at that time), Bryan McSwiney, approached two charitable foundations – the King Edward VII Fund for London and the Special Trustees of the Hospital – to see if they would jointly fund a senior position in the Hospital's Administration for a limited period of three years, to determine whether such a joint post was worthwhile. The post was funded and John Wyn Owen, an experienced hospital administrator, was appointed in 1972. Advantages to both the Research Unit and the Hospital Administration soon became evident. The administrator did not take over the management of the Research Unit but his presence sharpened the research performed and helped the administration to improve the hospital's management. A subsidiary benefit was that Mr Owen obtained a much better idea of the way researchers worked and what questions they could address. The researchers similarly benefited by a better understanding of what questions needed to be tackled as well as the timescale within which the administrator had to operate and would be able to use any findings or advice provided.

At the same time, the need for the hospital to coordinate its policies with the community became very evident from the results of the research. Informal contacts were inadequate, and thus a separate committee – the Committee on Community Care – was created in 1972 with representatives of the Local Authority (the Director of Public Health and staff, the Director of Social Services and staff), representatives of the local General Practitioners and of the Hospital, both administrators and clinicians. This Committee was managed by Mr Wyn Owen and served a very useful function in ensuring that services in Lambeth became more coherent and the gaps in service for particular groups, such as the disabled, were addressed.

The NHS was reorganised in 1974, the first such change since its foundation in 1948. The tripartite structure of hospital, local authority and general practice was dismantled and a unitary Area Health Authority created. The post, and independence, of the Clerk of the Governors disappeared and was replaced by the post of District Administrator. Similarly the Board of Governors disappeared and was replaced by the Area Health Authority, composed of representatives of the Local Authority, University (as we were a Teaching Hospital), hospital clinical staff such as consultants and nurses, and Trade Unions. The post of District Community Physician was created to replace the Local Authority's Director of Public Health; General Practice was administered by a subcommittee of the Area Health Authority. There are many descriptions of the changes and the problems and advantages they engendered. Many of the changes – particularly the concern for all health services to be coordinated and administered by one body – were in line with much that we had already been doing.

With the disappearance of the post of Clerk of the Governors, Mr McSwiney left to become Administrator of the Special Trustees and later to manage hospitals in the private sector at the behest of the Secretary of State, Barbara Castle. Mr Wyn Owen was appointed as District Administrator. The close links between the Research Unit and the District Health Administration were reinforced when as Research Unit Director I was elected SubDean of the Medical School and served on the District Management Team as university representative. This continued successfully for three years and the close links at local level between the research carried out and the health service administration undoubtedly improved both the research and the service. The District Administrator then moved to the private sector and my time on the District Management Team came to an end in 1977. With new people, new relationships, financial stringency and changes in research management in the Department of Health, the close and productive links were severed.

Mr Wyn Owen's subsequent career, first in the private sector, then as Director of NHS Wales, Director of New South Wales Health Authority (Australia) and finally as Secretary of the Nuffield Trust enabled him to play a different, but equally important, role in the encouragement of links between service and research. He was always sensitive to how research could be used most effectively.

I had also learnt a lot about how the service side, at local level, could use research and the topics we investigated in the Unit reflected this. I continued to play a role in the administration of local health services as a member of the District Health Authority, representing the university, and later as non-executive Director of a Health Authority (Gloucestershire). The close coordination between research and management/administration at local level for research concerned with changing operational structures and practice is enormously beneficial. Coordination with practitioners is also extremely important and is best achieved by the use of joint appointments and responsibilities. At St Thomas' this proved a good and very effective way to work and to improve the quality of both service and research at the operational level, although few other research units adopted this structure. This structure and way of working is, of course, much more difficult to achieve when the researchers are not embedded in a service organisation and a teaching hospital provides the ideal for this type of coordination.

Coordination at Central Level

Coordination and cooperation with central authorities or ministries is much more problematic. The central bodies see themselves as being in control and, as ultimate arbiters of what is to be funded and evaluated, may feel a need to keep researchers at a distance. When large amounts of money are being disbursed, it can be difficult to develop any degree of involvement. The crucial link between research and policy is the liaison officer and here there are at least two possible hazards. The first is that the liaison officer may not be trained in research and may have difficulty in understanding the particular project, the needs of the service and the personalities of those involved, and in managing the remit from above. The second is that in the UK the liaison officer in the Department of Health is a civil servant and may, therefore, have to move jobs and responsibilities if promoted or required in another department or sector, resulting in a loss of continuity. Problems of personality are always a possibility. For the relationship between researchers and liaison officers, the most troublesome of these arises when the latter consider their research expertise to be as good as, or better than, that of the researchers and try to impose their own ideas. Conversely, liaison officers can be invaluable in making researchers aware of opportunities, directing their efforts to where their strengths lie and alerting them to possible obstacles from the administration!

Most of the liaison officers we worked with were helpful, protective and pleasant. The vital beneficial role that can be played by a good liaison officer is well illustrated by the trial of multiphasic screening, described earlier. Dr J.M.G. (Max) Wilson, the responsible liaison officer for our Unit, had an interest in the evaluation of screening and had been to the US to review their methods. In 1968, with Dr G. Jungner, he published a short treatise on the subject for the World Health Organisation and was an acknowledged expert.[1]

The concept of multiphasic screening was superficially attractive in identifying individuals at a stage when their condition could be treated or reversed. Commercial companies, such as BUPA, were developing screening methods in the private sector. The Department of Health was aware that there would be pressure to introduce these into the NHS. At this time, in the late 1960s, health centres housing several general practitioners or several GP practices were being developed, and some were being built with facilities for investigation, such as X-ray and biochemistry tests. It was thus envisaged that multiphasic screening could be introduced into the NHS relatively easily and Dr Wilson appreciated the pressures to do so that would arise. We discussed the problem and agreed that it would be a fertile area for research. We decided that if the results were to be credible a proper randomised controlled trial would be required and we approached a number of the group practices who were to be located in the new purpose-built premises, without success. Eventually we contacted a GP principal, John Woodall, who had a history of research in general practice, and he and a neighbouring practice agreed to work with the Research Unit in undertaking a randomised controlled trial of multiphasic screening. The planning, execution and analysis was undertaken by individuals from the Unit and has already been discussed. In contrast to many current research commissions, the Department of Health accepted that this project would take at least eight years to reach any valid conclusions. It was one of the first projects that was truly multidisciplinary and involved not only doctors, epidemiologists, nurses and statisticians, but also economists.

The study was completed successfully. We were unable to show that multiphasic screening had any significant effect in reducing mortality or morbidity in the study group compared to the control group who received the normal medical care. We did show, however, that if routine multiphasic screening were to be introduced, the cost of the NHS would rise by about 10 per cent with no measurable benefit. As a result, to the chagrin of BUPA and other commercial organisations ready to jump on the bandwagon, it was decided that it should not be introduced. This was undoubtedly one of the major achievements of HSR – the amount of money saved paid for all the research we and others did many times over!

The pressure to introduce multiphasic screening – or periodic health examination as it is now more commonly known – has persisted.[2] We were fortunate that the Department of Health and politicians of the time were willing to resist populist and commercial pressures, and investigate and evaluate thoroughly. Unfortunately, things are now different and the Department has introduced so-called cardiovascular checks at the behest of politicians on the basis of economic modelling. This shows that the identification and treatment of certain parameters, such as levels of blood pressure and cholesterol, will improve life expectancy and reduce social costs, such as time off work. The process has been shown to be feasible but no randomised controlled trial has been carried out to demonstrate whether the cost and effort is worthwhile. Nor has any consideration been given as to whether population measures, such as a reduction of salt in the diet, would be more effective than the identification and labelling of individuals with certain risk characteristics.

Personal Coordination

Coordination between researchers and central bodies is enhanced when the researcher plays a role within the central body. This can be achieved by an exchange of personnel with the researcher seconded to work on a problem within the central department, or the administrator working in a research unit.

A second and most effective method of achieving this type of coordination is for the researcher to be a member of a relevant central committee, charged with evaluating or investigating a particular problem. I was involved in a number of Department of Health committees which had an impact on health policy. A good example of the role that a researcher can play in such a committee was the Resource Allocation Working Party (RAWP). The research and involvement of the St Thomas' Unit in this has been described in Chapter 6.

My role in this Working Party was to provide input on possible, reliable, routine information sources which could be used in the redistribution of resources. The Research Unit undertook a number of exploratory analyses to determine which data could best reflect regional morbidity variations – since at that time no such data were routinely available. The advice that mortality was a suitable indicator was accepted and used for many years.

Participation in a number of the committees concerned with environmental and behavioural hazards is easier to understand. Research studies provided knowledge of the effect on health of, for example, air pollution or of smoking cigarettes and the advice given was thus based on solid epidemiological evidence. The Department or Minister could accept or reject the findings but the research provided information based on scientific facts.

Another, slightly different, role that a researcher can fulfil is to provide advice and interpretation of scientific findings to government advisers. With the advent of Mrs Thatcher as Secretary of State for Education in 1970, a major change occurred in nutritional policy. Before her appointment, and since the start of the Second World War, the nutrition of mothers, babies, pre-school and schoolchildren had been supplemented by free school meals and milk. This had been introduced in view of the evidence of malnutrition in these groups before 1939. It had been continued as a social policy after the end of the Second World War. By the late 1960s there was an indication that the diet of mothers and children was adequate, and there were a number of studies indicating that the problem was now one of over-nutrition as shown by the occurrence of overweight and obesity, particularly in girls and lower social class groups. The cost of the nutritional supplementation was quite considerable (see Chapter 6).

The Conservative Government of 1970–1974 decided that this social policy was no longer necessary and that the money could be better used for the renovation and rebuilding of primary schools. It was also decided that a research programme of monitoring and surveillance would be established in order to warn if the change in policy had any harmful effect. Our Research Unit was given the task of establishing a national system of surveillance for schoolchildren and this has been described in detail.[3] It quickly became evident that the withdrawal of free school meals and milk did not have any significant deleterious effect (free school meals were still provided for the poor). The Labour Party, in its manifesto for the 1974 election, included the promise to restore free school milk and lunch to all primary schoolchildren. This policy was considered by the Cabinet in 1975–1976. The policy adviser to the

Secretary of State for Health at that time was Professor Brian Abel Smith who also served as Chairman of the Advisory Board of the St Thomas' Health Services Research Unit and discussed this policy with me. Our national surveillance of primary schoolchildren showed that the problem in this group was not under, but over-nutrition. At his request, I prepared a short briefing note for the Secretary of State and this was used by Mr David Ennals in Cabinet to help persuade his colleagues that the policy of nutritional supplementation should not be reinstated.

Thus HSR can and does play an important informal role in influencing both central and local policy and practice. Apart from influencing the treatment of individual patients, researchers involved in local policy decisions – for example on a medical or management committee – can play an important role. One of the skills of HSR is critical analysis of evidence. Managers are often faced with questions on whether to provide or abolish a particular service. These demands are frequently based on populist pressure. Researchers can advise about the adequacy of evidence for such action. This becomes even more important at higher levels of authority in decisions taken at ministerial level. Policy formulation is a complex procedure and this book cannot address such issues in any depth. But it should be acknowledged that most managers, health service administrators, civil servants, ministerial advisers and ministers are not trained in scientific principles or methods and often have little real knowledge of some of the factors concerned in making decisions or formulating health policy.

In my experience, the researcher involved at both formal and informal levels can play a crucial role – advising what are appropriate, feasible questions to ask, for example, for a piece of research. The research commissioner normally requires an answer to a general question, such as what resources are needed to provide treatment for a particular condition, or how can prevention policies best be substituted for treatment options. The researcher, if involved at an early stage, can help to refine such questions into researchable protocols. In the first case, for example, it would be necessary to define manpower needs and skills as well as facilities for treatment, investigation and follow-up. In the second, more complex, question of prevention versus treatment, the natural history of the condition under consideration and the long and short-term implications of a change in policy would be relevant.

The process of commissioning research requires a rigorous commissioning mechanism. The professional research organisations, such as the Research Councils, have developed expert mechanisms and individuals to do this. By contrast, in my experience, the Department of Health has, or at least had, a more haphazard approach in this area as several studies, such as those carried out by Kogan and colleagues, have demonstrated vividly.[4] Civil servants are mobile and tend to change posts and responsibilities frequently, and thus those involved in research management for short periods of time are unable to acquire the necessary expertise.

My own experience bears this out. In establishing the HSR Unit at St Thomas' we worked closely with the Office of the Chief Scientist (OCS) and related to the Chief Scientist, first Dr R.H.L. (Dick) Cohen from 1967–1973, then Sir Douglas Black 1973–1978, and the Senior Medical Administrator, Dr J.M.G. (Max) Wilson, as well as two professional administrators, John Cornish and Leslie Best. Cohen had been, for many years, at the Medical Research Council. Black was a skilled, respected medical researcher. Wilson had been an experienced clinician with a track record of research. Both they and we were interested in developing important, relevant research. We were dependent on each other. As researchers we wanted to have the means to do the research well, while the OCS was not only concerned with the acquisition of appropriate knowledge but was also anxious to perform a useful role which the Department of Health would respect. The professional administrators considered that their task was to ensure that these two complementary objectives were achieved within the bounds of administrative rules. The relationship was informal, friendly and helpful. The researchers were able to ask for help, when needed, whether for funds, equipment or access. The OCS and its staff felt free to ask us for advice – both on our own projects as well as on health service problems in general. Of course, although the relationship was informal, rules had to be followed and the results and quality of the research evaluated both explicitly and independently.

Over time this relationship between the OCS and researchers changed for various reasons. Personalities in the OCS and in the Department changed. The original senior figures retired and were replaced by individuals with less personal commitment to the development of HSR and less expertise in its disciplines. Structures became more bureaucratic and formalised, in part because the organisation had grown considerably, much more research was being commissioned and the Department had, to some extent, accepted the need for and existence of a research function. But the personal relationships and original informality disappeared and something important was lost. The researchers continued their work but there was a feeling that the commitment to HSR and the acceptance of its results were diminished. Financial resources for the NHS were under ever-increasing pressure and the relationship between research and service deteriorated.

This disillusion with research was epitomised by the correspondence between the Chief Scientist, myself, George Godber and R.H.L. (Dick) Cohen. The concern felt in medical research circles culminated in the Report of a House of Lords Committee on *Priorities for Medical Research* which concluded that the Department really did not care about research and was responsible for the loss of morale among researchers (see Chapter 7). The deliberations of this Committee resulted in a complete reform of research structure within the Department of Health, and the recognition of the importance of HSR to the nation and to a properly run health service.

An important and often overlooked method by which research can influence health policy is by the personal interaction of a researcher and health policy-maker. The generation and implementation of health policy at central level usually depends on the activities of senior grade administrative civil servants (assistant secretary level and above). It is these individuals who have access to Ministers and tend to be more trusted than the departmental medical officers who are often considered by ministers to be prisoners of their profession and are also sometimes considered less able than their non-medical counterparts.

The development of a meaningful, trusting relationship between a professional senior administrative civil servant and a researcher is an ideal which may be of immense help to both. The civil servant has considerable influence in the formulation of policy. Although policy is ultimately determined by the politically elected Minister, the Minister is usually not an expert in the field for which he or she is responsible. His or her view will be concerned with the political aspect, rather than the substantive content of a policy. Ministers change fairly frequently so the likelihood of a Minister developing in-depth knowledge in any area of responsibility is small. Within the British system the Minister has to rely on the civil servants within the Department to present a number of possible factual policy options for consideration based on their own expertise, what they have gleaned from their reading and from discussion with their colleagues and others.

As a group of health service researchers, we often had difficulties with both field and central managers and administrators, both in the design of appropriate research capable of answering their questions as well as in the implementation of results. This was understandable. Our priorities were to ask meaningful questions, to carry out the research and to implement findings. Research may also reveal politically unwelcome findings – for example, the services provided are quite inadequate for a particular risk group such as the deprived, but appropriate for others, such as the relatively affluent middle classes, or that a particular service is inadequate. One such example is the service provided for addiction to drugs such as cocaine or cannabis. While the affluent middle classes are able to afford the time off work when receiving treatment, this is rarely the situation among the more deprived in whom addiction may be far more common. The more affluent will also know of and ask for such services – the less well-off rarely know or do!

As we were a stable group involved in a variety of health service issues, we gradually developed a relationship based on openness and trust with one or two of the senior administrators in the Department of Health. We were made aware of issues that might fruitfully be explored, as well as those where research scrutiny might be less acceptable. We, in exchange, were able to provide independent advice to illuminate a number of health policy areas. It was crucial for both sides to be able to rely on complete confidentiality. This relationship was of benefit to us as researchers and undoubtedly helped in the development of sound health policies.

TIMESCALE

A recurring and inevitable problem with most HSR commissioned by governmental agencies and departments is the timescale. Politicians work to an electoral timetable with a general election normally every four to five years and want results before they lose power or change jobs. Unfortunately, sound HSR is rarely possible within this sort of timescale. Setting up a trial or a survey is likely to take a minimum of several months and, with the present need for approval from ethical and medical committees, this is often extended to at least a year.

Recruitment of adequate numbers of individuals or patients for the study might take up to two years, followed by suitable follow-up, evaluation, analysis and writing up for reporting and publication. All this implies that any reasonable investigations will take five years or more to be concluded satisfactorily as illustrated by the studies previously described.

This timescale, essential to the integrity of the research, is often unacceptable to the politicians and thus a variety of other strategies have to be considered as described below:

● Ideally the commissioner of the research will persuade his or her current Minister that certain studies are needed for the general good rather than for political reasons. This approach depends on both the skill of the administrator in convincing the Minister and the willingness of the latter to accept the advice.

- The researchers and commissioners of research (including the Research Councils or the Departmental body) have planned the research in such a way that it will answer questions in the future rather than immediately. This depends on wisdom and cooperation on both sides.
- Commissioners of research abandon the collection of new data and persuade the researchers to base their research on available routine data sources. This is very attractive, particularly with the current plethora of routine data collected for management or audit or other purposes. Commissioners, as well as the researchers, must be content to accept the deficiencies of routine data such as incompleteness, inaccuracies, observer variability and lack of ability to be certain of appropriate denominators. This may be due to lack of knowledge of the sources of error – but it may also be due to willingness to accept errors because of the much lower cost and rapidity of getting an answer. It is unfortunate that more and more HSR is done by analysis of routine sources rather than primary data collection. It is even more unfortunate that researchers do not explore the possible sources of error in routine data sources (such as patient records) which could easily be done on small samples to give some idea of validity.
- With the increasing availability of computers and the development of modelling techniques, many current policies are developed on the basis of predictions from computer mathematical models. This is, of course, the dominant method of economic analysis and it is not surprising that, with the increasing influence of economists in the health service field, this has come about. But when such techniques are used in health services the lessons of economic models used in commerce and finance are often forgotten. The assumptions and model developed are bound to affect the result. Thus models of our economy developed by the Bank of England, the Treasury and individual consultancies often give quite different results on such matters as future inflation or growth of debt. In such an area policy-makers develop a degree of scepticism, and take into account the different scenarios depicted in the decisions they make. In health, however, different rules seem to apply. Recent examples are the development of a statistical model for the number of deaths to be expected from BSE in 1998. The modellers did give an idea of the variability of their predictions, but there has been little public comment that the lowest limit of the predictions is what occurred

(less than 200 rather than several thousands). The Department of Health and Ministers do not seem to have accepted the fallibility of such models. Models were also developed in relation to the expected swine flu outbreak, and, on the basis of these, decisions were taken on how many doses of anti-flu drugs should be purchased. In the event, far fewer cases and deaths occurred than predicted. The emphasis on mathematical models came at the expense of setting up more effective systems of disease surveillance based on actually devising methods of disease identification and containment as had been done during previous outbreaks. Even more recently, 2008–2009, cardiovascular checks are being introduced in general practice based on economic models of how many cases of cardiovascular disease could be prevented by the identification and treatment of individuals with raised blood pressure and cholesterol. Little attention has been paid to past experience in properly organised randomised controlled trials which did not show any benefit in terms of morbidity and mortality for such screening procedures. The much more effective population measures such as reduction of salt and fat intake have been ignored.

● Over the last 20 years there has been increasing turmoil in the NHS. Between 1948 and 1974 there was stability in the structure and organisation – which was reflected in the type and quantity of HSR studies. The 1974 reorganisation of the NHS was the result of a large number of reports written by experts, usually from within the service – for example, John Fry, the BMA, Robert Hunter – although, of course, there were also a number of Ministerial Committees, such as the Crossman Committee on Function of Regions. Since 1974 there have been innumerable reorganisations and the number has increased since 1990. One of the major characteristics of these changes has been the relative neglect of NHS professionals in their design. The changes have usually been politically motivated – for example, the purchaser-provider split, Foundation Trusts and so on. Ministers have tended to involve their own political advisers in the design and implementation and there has been little, if any, involvement of expert health services researchers or staff. These changes have had an influence on the type of HSR that has been commissioned. Most of the changes in structure and organisation have been based on descriptive documents, often of an analytical type, but none on actual field experiments or observations: at best, lessons or findings have been based on the experience in other countries. This method of exploring alternative ways to deliver health services has also been adopted frequently in the consideration of less major changes in health service delivery, such as the management of waiting lists, personal 'health trainers', use of nurses or pharmacists instead of doctors in the delivery of some services. These techniques obviously take much less time to execute and can be done within the lifetime of a Parliament but are frequently evidence-free. The expertise of HSR built up over the past 40 years is thus neglected because of political expediency.

- There has been an increasing tendency in the NHS to use management consultants to analyse, describe and solve problems, but in June 2010 it was stated that the bill for management consultants to the Department of Health was almost £500 million, much more than is spent on HSR!

In the late 1960s and early 1970s management consultants, such as McKinsey, were used in the period leading up to the 1974 NHS reorganisation. This work was supervised by committees of NHS experts who were able to comment on and guide the process. They were used partly because at that time there was little health service expertise in organisational change. There was only one HSR Unit at Brunel University led by Professor Jacques with any relevant experience. The consultants were also able to deploy rapidly sufficient numbers of analysts to enable progress to be made in the required time. However, over time, the use of management consultant firms has increased very considerably. Ministers and managers like them partly because they work fast, they can deploy analysts far more rapidly than any university or research unit, and they do what they are told. They also provide the required answers without any of the concerns with validity that beset researchers, and their reports and results are confidential – they do not need to be open to public scrutiny or publication.

Some of the management consultancy groups involved include ex-academic HSR researchers in search of employment and good financial rewards. It is unfortunate that government neglects to provide sufficient support to academic HSR to enable the discipline to perform the function commissioned from private, for-profit organisations. Some of the problems tackled by management consultants are well done but many are not. This may in part be the result of political pressures and time constraints but it is also very often due to the lack of critical evaluation of the methods and conclusions and unwillingness to consider alternative solutions. The need to develop so many different NHS organisation models, over the past 20 years, is partly because of the inadequacy of the analysis of the problems of health service delivery, and the absence of evidence in many cases of the solutions proposed and implemented.

EVALUATION OF RESEARCH

The methods for evaluation are no different in HSR to those used in any form of research. Research commissioned or investigator-initiated needs to be submitted in the form of a protocol containing a hypothesis, the methods to be used in the investigation including appropriate analysis, the population to be investigated and methods of dissemination. The real problem with HSR is that almost every example is multidisciplinary and, therefore, involves a combination of clinical, epidemiological, social science and statistical methods. When HSR was first started it was unusual for these disciplines to be equally represented in a research proposal – or even all the methods required to be applied in the proposals submitted. Part of this was due to the shortage of researchers in the relevant disciplines, and also because the discipline in its infancy was not considered attractive to experts in the required fields. But it was also partly because the topics required multidisciplinary working, a methodology not common in the 1960s, when most investigations concerned only one discipline. In addition, those attracted to multidisciplinary work lost status in their own discipline and thus promotion in their parent discipline might be difficult. But above all such work requires training and trust in collaborators involved in tackling a problem.

At the beginning of the organisation of HSR there was a scheme to fund investigator-initiated small grant proposals. The Assessment Committee, of which I was a member, was made up of individuals from all the disciplines. Every member judged each proposal and the final score formed the criterion by which the grant was assessed. The Chairman of the Committee kept a tally of the scores by each member, and their comments on the relevant component of the proposal. It was rapidly appreciated that the epidemiologists tended to be most critical of the epidemiological/statistical grant applications, but viewed social science applications far more favourably then the social scientists – and vice versa. Thus we had to develop a methodology of assessment which took into account our different perspectives so that we could trust each other to make a fair and objective judgement.

The assessment of the work of an HSR Unit was more complex. Research Units had not only to navigate the original grant approval for their projects but were usually assessed at intervals, usually five years, on their total programme. The Units were funded on the basis of a five-year rolling contract. Each Unit was funded to undertake a defined programme – it did not need to submit grant proposals for each research project within the defined programme. Each Unit was expected to be willing to undertake research in its area of expertise commissioned by the Department of Health who would provide additional resources if needed. Each Unit could also undertake work within its remit on its own initiative if agreed by the Department. The advantage of this was that the Unit could recruit researchers who had relative job security and could thus build up expertise and develop a body of HSR researchers and our Unit at St Thomas' was also specifically empowered to recruit young researchers for training. Earlier in the book, I have described the methods we developed to ensure that the quality of our research met the standards of each of the parent disciplines. Certainly the ability to recruit young, able, enthusiastic researchers and train them in multidisciplinary research paid off. The number of professors, consultants and senior researchers trained at St Thomas' was considerable, ranging from the Chief Statistician of the UK Office of National Statistics to Professors in Epidemiology, Sociology and Medical Statistics in many UK, US and Australian Universities as well as the Chief Economist at the World Health Organisation.

The evaluation of the work of a Research Unit was difficult. Usually the Unit was assessed by a group of four or five scientists from a mix of disciplines, as well as representatives of the Department of Health. Before any assessment visit the Unit had to prepare a compendium of the research done in the previous five years as well as its future programme of work. These papers had to be read and evaluated by the visitors. The Unit then had to present its work orally to the visitors in a meeting of about four to six hours with subsequent discussion. The visitors gave a report of their evaluation, usually in preliminary form at the end of the visit, and then prepared a final written report. This report was transmitted to the Unit, who were able to comment on it before it was submitted to the appropriate Department of Health Chief Scientist Committee for a decision on further funding.

The timing of visits was such that the contract for the Unit usually had two more years to run, thus enabling both the Department of Health and the Unit to make appropriate arrangements for the staff in the event of a decision to terminate.

As both a recipient of such research evaluation visits as well as a member and Chairman of some evaluations, I can attest to the stressful and difficult nature of these assessments. The evaluation of multidisciplinary research is always more difficult than the evaluation of work in an individual discipline. Compromises in design and analysis of such research must often be made if it is to answer a particular question. Judgement is thus required of the weight to be placed on the importance of any one aspect in the solution of a problem. Far more fraught, however, is the judgement of the research unit work on an applied problem. There could be conflict between the perspectives of the commissioner (the Department of Health), the researchers and the assessors – particularly if they included individuals responsible for the delivery of a service, whether in a hospital or in the community. The Department of Health were often at odds with the providers of services in the period 1970–1990, the academics were frequently dubious about some of the questions the Department of Health were posing and were sometimes dismissive of the concerns that the providers raised. The visiting academic assessors could also, at times, consider that the research carried out was unimaginative or sloppy, often because of their own ignorance of service needs and constraints.

Two examples illustrate the difficulty. Our evaluation of the work of a Unit concerned with the management of mental handicap showed the inadequacy of knowledge on how to treat such patients by both the visiting scientists and the representatives of the Department of Health. In reviewing a Unit involved in the collection and analysis of general practice activity, the visiting research assessors were disappointed by the unimaginative analyses undertaken – but had not appreciated that simple descriptive data had been requested by the Department of Health. The Unit's resources were inadequate to provide analyses of greater sophistication in which the Department was in any case profoundly uninterested.

Thus these research assessments depended to a great extent on the wisdom of the visiting Chairman, the interpretation of the evaluation by the Department of Health, and, of course, the OCS.

PUBLICATION AND CONFIDENTIALITY

When the original contracts between HSR researchers and Units were drawn up, in the mid-to-late1960s, the expectation was that all research undertaken would be published. The Medical Research Council, Department of Health and charities supporting such research encouraged publication in peer-reviewed journals and books as long as acknowledgement was made of the funding source. All research funders expected to receive a draft copy of the research report before submission for publication. The Department of Health stated explicitly that any proposed publication should be submitted to them, giving them one month to comment. The researchers were free to accept or reject the comments or amendments from the Department of Health but if they were rejected, a further one month's notice had to be given before the report appeared in print. Researchers considered these to be entirely reasonable conditions and the comments received often added value to the proposed publication.

With the increase in the number of HSR investigations and change in both the political atmosphere and the confidence of research management, this arrangement began to falter in the mid-1980s. The spark for this could have been the report from a highly competent research unit on a survey of chiropody services that showed the inadequacy of provision. The Conservative Government, at that time, was very sensitive to publication of critical reports in view of the reduction in expenditure on public services, including the NHS. At the same time the Health Education Council (a government-supported body) published material critical of the increase in poverty and the growing social divide between rich and poor. Many academics involved in HSR, both in medicine and social science, were vociferous in their condemnation of the government's policies.

As a result of this turmoil, the Department of Health endeavoured to stop the publication of research they had funded or were currently funding if the administrative staff and politicians felt that the findings could be interpreted as criticism of government policies. The researchers were united in their opposition to any inhibition of the publication of research results – the source of the funds for the research was considered irrelevant. Ministers and their staff came under great pressure to inhibit the publication of critical research, aided by the populist press and some very right wing politicians. The St Thomas' Unit was in the fortunate position of having a contract with explicit conditions on rights to publish. Of course we had a rolling contract which could be terminated but its nature was such that we always had five years' security – enough time for a change in attitudes. Other researchers, particularly new starters, did not have such binding contracts and attempts were made to introduce censorship capabilities. Universities, as well as individuals, became very concerned with this governmental interference. Politicians were lobbied – and the House of Lords Select Committee on Priorities for Medical Research was scathing in its condemnation of any form of censorship. Fortunately the Department of Health and the Chief Scientist saw sense and the policy on publication resumed its former status. Nonetheless since 1990 the conditions for publication by researchers have become more stringent under the guise of Crown Copyright! As far as I am aware, however, no sound academic research critical of any health or social policy has been prevented from publication. On the contrary, most research proposals now require the applicant to describe the dissemination strategies in some detail. It has been recognised that many useful research results have remained unknown or disregarded because of the inadequacies of dissemination – including the practice of publishing only in academic journals, the preferred academic route!

Linked to the problems of publication of research findings has been data protection and confidentiality. Rules of data protection are very important and we were often at fault in not paying sufficient attention to this. There was an example of this in the St Thomas' Research Unit in the 1960s during the studies on health care needs in Lambeth that entailed a private census of a random sample of households. This census was done by fieldworkers whom we employed, and the data were tabulated and analysed by our statisticians.

While this was being done, the Clerk of the Governors of St Thomas' received a complaint from an elderly lady living in the catchment area of the census. She had received a letter from an insurance agent asking her to take out a policy and stating that her name had been suggested by a St Thomas' employee. She remembered that she had received a visit from one of our fieldworkers and I was asked to investigate. We had collected her personal details and these had been tabulated and analysed by one of our statistical assistants. We rapidly identified the individuals involved in handling these data and the statistical assistant admitted to providing an insurance agent with the name and details of individuals who might benefit from taking out an insurance policy. The assistant was immediately dismissed. But we were also at fault in assuming that researchers involved in our study would conform to the medically accepted practice of confidentiality. As a result of this episode we introduced a simple document which had to be read, signed and adhered to by all members of the Research Unit. No further breach occurred.

There is now a much stricter set of conditions for researchers involved in data collection and on how the data can be used. To many researchers these rules have become very restrictive and have greatly increased the bureaucracy involved in field investigations. It has been forgotten that participation in any field study is voluntary. There must be rules of behaviour, and suitable sanctions, but it is doubtful that all the regulations which now exist serve a useful purpose.

The increasing difficulties in doing field research – as a result of various obstacles such as cost, having to obtain approval to use a questionnaire, reluctance of individuals to participate in research or to answer questions – has meant that an increasing number of HSR investigations rely on available data-sets which have not been specifically tailored to answer a hypothesis but that do contain information that can be used in answering a given question. Unfortunately, many of these studies neglect the possibilities of error since the data have usually been collected for administrative purposes and do not necessarily undergo adequate checks on validity or sources of variation and were not primarily designed to answer a given HSR question. Large population data-sets, usually collected for national statistical purposes, such as general household surveys, are increasingly being used. These have normally been tested for data validity – but often it is forgotten that responses to national surveys such as this suffer from problems of inadequate response rates – less important for a national survey, but possibly crucial for an HSR study. Furthermore, the number in a specific possible 'at risk' group is too small for any useful generalisation. Thus the tasks of HSR have become more difficult than in the past.

CONCLUSION

This chapter has attempted to illuminate some of the complexities of HSR. Basic or experimental research is simpler. A question or problem requires an appropriate protocol with suitable methodology. The investigation needs to be executed to an acceptable standard, analysed and reported. HSR needs all this but, in addition, must navigate organisational, political and human obstacles which often mean that the best design cannot be used. It is also essential that those undertaking HSR have real knowledge of the health service and how it works. Only if all these criteria are met is it likely to provide useful guidance.

REFERENCES

1   Wilson, J.M.G. and Jungner, G. (1968). *Principles and Practice of Screening for Disease*. Geneva: World Health Organisation.
2   Holland, W. (2009). Periodic health examination – a brief history and critical assessment. *Eurohealth*, **15**, 16–20.
3   Rona, R.J. and Chinn, S. (1999). *The National Study of Health and Growth*. Oxford: Oxford University Press.
4   Kogan, M., Korman, N. and Henkel, M. (1980). *Government Commissioning of Research: a Case Study*. London: Department of Government Brunel University.

9. Conclusions

I have tried in this book to describe the field of HSR and consider its background, methods and applications. It has been written very much from a personal perspective in the hope that lessons for the future can be drawn.

IMPORTANCE OF EVIDENCE AND EVALUATION

Medicine has always been considered as an art as well as a science and the best medicine is certainly both. Until the 1950s the criteria for diagnosis and treatment of a condition were usually based on pathophysiological knowledge and experiments, and the past experience of the doctor involved in a particular case. The demonstration of the effectiveness of streptomycin in the treatment of pulmonary tuberculosis in randomised controlled trials, carried out by the Medical Research Council group, led by Sir Austin Bradford Hill and published in 1948, changed all that[1] and evidence-based medicine was born.

Today it is expected that the effectiveness of any treatment will have been formally assessed before it is introduced. In the UK, the National Institute for Clinical Excellence is charged with the assessment of the cost-effectiveness of all new drugs before they are prescribed in the NHS and also provides reviews of and guidelines for all forms of management of particular conditions such as, for example, stroke, obesity or high blood pressure.

The acceptance of formal, systematic evaluation of possible treatment and management of diseases and conditions is also of relatively recent origin. It was first stimulated by Archie Cochrane's 1972 Rock Carling Lecture entitled *Effectiveness and Efficiency: Random Reflections on Health Services.*[2] Since the early 1990s, further stimulus has been provided by Sir Ian Chalmers through the Cochrane collaboration.[i]

---

[i] An international collaboration of researchers who conduct systematic reviews of health care randomised controlled trials and publish the results in the Cochrane Library.

HSR has played a major part in a change in the culture in medicine in emphasising the need for and acceptance of the findings of proper evaluation of past, current and future practice – for example, in studies of short-stay surgery or the value of screening. But it is remarkable how resistant policy-makers, both professional and political, have been to the need for and use of research in changing the practice, organisation and structure of health services. In the UK as elsewhere, this may be partly because health policy has traditionally been dominated by civil servants and politicians with a non-scientific background who may resist encroachment by specialists into what they regard as their territory. But the 'political' nature of health services and the prevention, treatment and rehabilitation of disease must be fully understood and, if HSR is to fulfil its full potential in the planning, delivery and evaluation of health services, it must have entry into these domains. It would be pointless to deny the existence of the tensions between politics and research but lessons can and should be learnt from past experience.

The research group must have the vision to be able to identify fruitful areas for research and methods of working and, most importantly, must be able to consider the potential applications of the results. The client or customer is a crucial component, whether the end user is, for example, a clinician or the commissioner from a Health Authority or the Department of Health. If there is no formal commissioner, the researcher must consider the potential market for research that is being planned or submitted. Relationships between customers and researchers can be fraught. Most customers within a research-service structure are repre-sented by a liaison officer who will deal officially with the research group and this can lead to difficulties that have to be handled diplomati-cally – the best liaison officer is a treasure, the worst a nightmare.

Liaison officers in the Office of the Chief Scientist (OCS) were medically qualified – former GPs or consultants in public health services – or social scientists or basic scientists. They were all civil servants, often drafted into the OCS for a limited period and then returned to their administrative/policy roles. By contrast, liaison officers in the Medical Research Council, of similar background and training, were career research managers.

An example of excellence in liaison was seen in our study of screening with Dr J.M.G. (Max) Wilson (Chapter 6). The studies on disability (Chapter 6) had greater problems since the liaison officer was not as expert in the field.

Researchers often prefer a direct relationship with the customer – for example, the administrator or clinician responsible for the service on which research is being focused or the civil servant or politician who is directly or indirectly interested in a particular research project. Experience has proved that the liaison officer may have misunderstood the problem to be investigated or may have more expertise and a wish to impose the method used and interpretation of the findings. The researchers, on the other hand, may claim fuller knowledge of the research agenda and how to handle it. There is no easy solution to these difficulties but it is important to be aware that they can exist and must be dealt with. The development of trust and a belief that each player is doing their best and is being honest and forthright in explaining or describing any difficulties arising during the conduct of the research are perhaps the most crucial attributes of the relationship between researcher, liaison officer and customer.

The abilities and skills of the health services researcher are of fundamental importance in this multidisciplinary field. It is essential that the methods used in any study, whether observational or experimental, are of the highest standard and acknowledged as such by those in the relevant disciplines. All studies in HSR must be aware of possible problems such as observer variability, inadequate response rates, representativeness of the population studied, appropriate statistical or economic measures or time–area–subject variability.

In most cases the customers will want results quickly and may try to persuade researchers to use less stringent methodology in the interests of speed. Few political or administrative agencies are prepared to accept lengthy timescales – the electoral cycle of a maximum of five years in the UK often drives investigations. Some service organisations will accept a longer-term timescale and may seek the necessary funds from a research council which is less prone to political pressures. But this can present other problems – particularly of the willingness of the council to fund applied research, often considered of lesser merit than basic research.

Researchers must also be aware of the constraints of time in the delivery of results. A prime example of this came in 1965–1966 in the course of an investigation to estimate the number of intensive nursing care beds needed in the rebuild of St Thomas' Hospital.

A methodologically sound study design was devised in which each current ward was visited on a regular basis over one year, in order to avoid seasonal biases. The visits were timed so that a ward was not visited on the same day each week, and a scheme designed whereby the assessment of need for intensive nursing care was assessed objectively and related to the diagnosis. The observations took one year and the analysis a further six months.[3] By the time we presented the results to management, however, the decision on the number of beds required had already been taken by the architect and builders – based on a one month operational research study included in building guidance. The two studies came to the same conclusion on the number of beds needed in relation to the total size of the new hospital. Our longer but more methodologically sound study could be used in modelling the number of beds required in relation to changes in 'case-mix' since we had details of the diagnoses of patients. But that was its only advantage. This study illustrated that, in HSR intended to influence practical operational decisions, it is important to be aware of the timescale in which decisions will have to be made and to recognise that 'perfect' epidemiological studies are not necessarily the only way to tackle a particular problem.

Our experience in this investigation also illustrates the importance of dialogue with other health professionals. Although we worked with two very experienced nurses (one a future Chief Nursing Officer), we did not involve any clinical medical staff in the design or execution of the study and relied entirely on the nursing assessments. When the study was presented to the medical staff, it was severely criticised for under-estimating the need for intensive nursing care beds. They considered that with clinical advances more rather than fewer beds would be needed. More fundamental, however, was our failure to take account of infection control necessitating the isolation of patients with infected wounds.

The ability and expertise of the research team were not in question but the outcomes of this and other studies underline the need to involve clinicians or other personnel in the design, conduct, analysis and application of any HSR project. A key research role must be to act as a bridge between those concerned with policy formulation and those charged with implementing any new practice or change in current procedures. Too often, senior policy-makers fail to involve front-line staff of *all* disciplines and grades in discussions on possible changes and in formulating the questions that research needs to ask to evaluate existing practices or explore new models.

RESEARCH PRIORITIES

Every commissioning body develops a strategy for deciding on their research programme. Some will specify their priorities in great detail and will establish elaborate machinery for consultation and involvement of consumers, providers and managers. But this machinery does not always work effectively and problems can and do arise. Some of the more common of these are described below.

1. Continuity

   Individuals in positions of authority in any organisation commissioning or funding research inevitably change and there can be a lack of continuity and stability in priorities that will affect long-term projects.

2. Strategies

   Specification of research priorities in great detail may seem attractive superficially but is rarely helpful. Broad strategies – such as the prevention of heart disease or the substitution of manpower skills in the treatment of a patient group – are far more helpful. It is part of the task of the HSR team to plan the detail of the project.

3. Research interest

   A keen interest in the problem under investigation is a crucial prerequisite for good research and the researcher should understand how any results will be applied or improve knowledge. Quality of research must be the aim and this implies that the researchers must care about the work they are doing and be proud of the results.

4. Accommodation and funding

   On a practical level, accommodation and funding must be available for researcher-initiated as well as commissioned research. Researchers themselves are often most aware of the work that needs to be done and researcher-initiated studies can provide the stimulus to long-term commitment to a particular topic or area with beneficial results.

5. Solutions

   Researchers and research commissioners must recognise that perfect solutions or methods may not be practicable or attainable and must agree to accept solutions that are credible, valid and acceptable.

DATA

Much current HSR involves the use of databases collected for a variety of clinical or administrative purposes. This has a number of advantages – the data are readily available and are usually based on very large numbers or populations. But there are also serious disadvantages. The researcher has no control of the data available and these may not be exactly what are required for the particular purpose. There has often been little concern with validity or accuracy and the possibility of observer-subject variability may have been neglected. There is no control either over the response rate or completeness of the data and this may result in a highly selected population and other potential sources of bias.

On the other hand, the fieldwork involved in data collection specifically for a particular investigation is time-consuming and expensive. It will certainly be more reliable and checks can be introduced to reduce observer variability or observer-subject variation – as, for example, as in the recording of blood pressure – but time and cost constraints may make it impossible.

I much regret the demise of the tradition of fieldwork in the gathering of population/patient/provider information. But I am even more concerned that few researchers have developed essential measures of quality control in the collection of routine administrative or clinical data. It is extremely rare today to find routine data-sets subjected to measures of quality such as duplicate measurements by questioning a small random sample or checks against a reference sample.

The problems of response rate or selection of sample also seem to be neglected. In the past, it was expected that 90 per cent of a target population would be included in a study. Many researchers now are satisfied with a response rate of 50–60 per cent. More worrying still, in terms of research rigour, is that few take the necessary measures to determine how 'selected' this 50–60 per cent is. Intensive, concentrated study of a small proportion of the 40–50 per cent of non-respondents could achieve the knowledge necessary to judge the reliability of the results obtained.

DESIGN

Study design is of critical importance in any research study. Appropriate design will take account of the use to be made of the results and thus the degree of accuracy required. This in turn will influence the size of the investigation.

In general, researchers are interested in studies that will be considered scientifically sound and provide a reliable and statistically significant result. But researchers need to be aware that the 'perfect' study may not produce a result of practical relevance to administrators or policy-makers. This was illustrated very clearly in the intensive care beds study described above and underlines the gap between researchers striving for excellence and scientific credibility, and administrators and policy-makers looking for reliable, practical and timely research advice.

Researchers must be able to bridge this gap. Perhaps the most usual way to do this is to be content with a study design that may be less scientifically robust but that will provide competent results within a reasonable timescale.

A less than perfect study design, however, may have two major unfortunate consequences. First, the commissioners of the research may be able more easily to dismiss the findings if they do not agree with them on the pretext that it was an inadequate study. An example of this was the finding of increasing obesity in schoolchildren in the late 1980s and early 1990s in the National Study of Health and Growth (Chapter 6). Second, an external scientific assessor may question the scientific adequacy of the study and reject it on this basis. Our research on avoidable mortality (Chapter 6) was regarded with suspicion by assessors, partly because of the conditions selected for study but also because of the lack of sophisticated statistical analysis. These possible scenarios must be considered by researchers and commissioners at the start of the study and both parties must agree to accept the consequences of a particular design.

When a particular research problem is presented, consideration must be given on how it can best be solved. For much of HSR direct observations or experiments will not be feasible – because of time constraints, funding or unwillingness to accept research findings. It may be necessary, therefore, to choose a suitable proxy measure to answer the question. In the determination of relative need for health services and the allocation of resources to authorities, for example, we suggested the use of age-standardised mortality ratios for specific causes on the grounds that areas with high mortality rates were likely to have greater need for health services than areas with low rates. The statistical data for morbidity that was available nationally – for example, sickness absence rate or the results of health surveys – might have been better, but this data had other disadvantages such as not being available for all age groups or in sufficient numbers to be statistically robust. All such data sources were highly correlated but mortality data covered the whole country, were reliable and acceptable and, most importantly, were available when required. In addition, they did not show large annual variations and could thus be used reliably for funding allocation.[4]

In our work on trying to determine the health care needs of the Lambeth population (Chapter 6), the prevalence, severity and treatment received by a random sample of the population for chronic cardio-respiratory disease, skin disease, disability and peptic ulcer were measured. These four conditions were considered as a proxy for health care in general and rather better than utilisation data that represented demand rather than need. Thus we used these as indicators rather than attempting an unrealistic study of the total picture.

The use of indicators in HSR is well accepted by most researchers although it can be and often is questioned by the customer. Researchers, therefore, must be involved with commissioners of research at all levels, both to devise appropriate methods for investigation *and* to advise on what can and cannot be done. Researchers must also consult those who will be expected to implement any policy arising from the research results. Practitioners, such as doctors, nurses and managers, have the essential practical knowledge about the delivery of current services as well as the likely effects of possible changes. It is crucial that all involved in the research process – researchers, political and administrative commissioners, liaison officers and practitioners – must be able and willing to discuss the problems and possible solutions in order to change current practice or introduce a new service or method.

Thus the involvement of practising clinicians in the design and execution of HSR is essential although this may mean that the most rigorous study design cannot be used. The evaluation of renal lithotripsy – a new non-invasive method of removal of renal stones – provides an example of this (Chapter 6). The conduct of a randomised controlled trial of the new lithotripter machinery compared to percutaneous removal of the renal stone was not accepted. The clinicians involved did not consider that it was fair for patients to be randomly allocated to a non-invasive versus a minimally invasive procedure. So a paired comparison of patients subjected to these procedures had to be used. The resistance of the clinicians to a randomised controlled trial was also influenced by the fact that percutaneous nephrolithotomy was only practised in one or two hospitals and not in the one hospital that had a lithotripter. Thus, random allocation of patients to the two treatments could have entailed patients referred for treatment in one institution being treated in another.

This study also showed that willingness to adopt new methods of treatment or management on the basis of objective investigation may be dismissed, both by practitioners and managers. The results of the study showed that lithotripsy was more expensive and no more effective than percutaneous nephrolithotomy but this did not discourage the administrators from buying more lithotripters. Eventually, there were more machines than required so the criteria for the treatment of renal stones was changed and smaller stones were treated much more often. A scenario of 'machines in search of stones' was the result! This example illustrates the fact that persuasive clinicians with a plausible story can be more effective than the results of a respectable although not perfect HSR study.

Modifications to the NHS are often taken for political reasons rather than being based on factual findings and there are two recent examples of this.

The current proposals for major change in the organisation of the NHS by introducing GP commissioning build on past Conservative Party policy on GP fundholding at the beginning of the 1990s. Fundholding was evaluated and the changes were shown to have been of marginal benefit.[5-8] In spite of this, the current Coalition Government plans to introduce radical changes in the NHS structure and function by making GP consortia responsible for at least 80 per cent of the commissioning of health services. There has been little preparation or evaluation of the cumulative effects of this on specialist services or an acknowledgement that a change from the consideration of need for NHS services may be replaced by demand.

The second recent example of a health policy introduced without adequate consideration is that of 'Health Checks' in England for all individuals aged 40 years and over. The intention is to provide a structured risk assessment in general practice for coronary heart disease, cerebrovascular disease and type II diabetes. Assessment was done on the basis of a number of complex models that showed that the programme would produce significant benefits. This policy is being introduced in spite of the findings of a randomised controlled trial of multiphasic screening in general practice that failed to show any reduction in either mortality or measures of morbidity.[9] A review of periodic health examinations has confirmed the lack of a benefit of such a strategy in other studies[10] and the UK National Screening Committee considers that these health checks do not meet its stringent criteria.

It is unfortunate that national policy-makers rarely accept that policies should not be implemented simultaneously in the whole country. It seems obvious that, with proper design, evaluation could be done by rigorous study of a new policy in the area in which it is first introduced – essentially, that new policies should be implemented in a planned order. Policies could then be modified on the basis of the evaluation in the first area before being implemented elsewhere. The use of large, experimental pilots, with proper evaluation, is not very common in this country and institutional memories of past policy evaluations are poor if not entirely absent!

PUBLICATION

All researchers seek to have their findings published but in recent years publication rights have been the subject of some controversy. Research on the effect of drugs has been particularly contentious. Drug companies who sponsor a trial often attempt to influence the publication of the results and researchers in this field have understandably become wary of this. Journals now also expect authors to list all possible areas of conflict of interest such as funding of the trial, consultancy, payment for journeys and lectures so that readers can judge whether it is likely that the results have been influenced or biased.

Similar concerns can arise in the publication of the results of HSR. When this kind of research was first supported by the Department of Health, the contract included a statement that the results of the research would be published in an appropriate scientific journal. The researchers were expected to acknowledge the source of the research funds and to show the proposed publication to the Department of Health for comment before submission. Any comments had to be made within a defined period of time, in the case of our Unit one month. The comments were intended to improve the proposed publication but researchers had the right to reject them as long as the Department was informed.

There were two main reasons for this system. The first was to enable the Department to be prepared for any public comment on the published paper. The second was to make the researcher aware of any knowledge the Department had not previously disclosed and to know in advance the reactions of the Department to the proposed publication.

Throughout my active research career we had no problems with this procedure. In the mid-1980s, however, problems with publication rights arose. It has been suggested that these began when a health services researcher published the findings of a study that was critical of chiropody services and invoked the displeasure of the then Secretary of State for Health. The freedom to publish was considered very important to researchers who became concerned that the Department of Health was trying to restrict this. The House of Lords Enquiry on *Priorities in Medical Research: Volume 1 Report* (paragraph 4.15)[11] commented as follows:

> particularly in relation to public health research the committee stress the importance of the right to publish in maintaining independence and the standards of research. They were not entirely reassured by the Minister of Health's statement about the revision of DHSS research contracts in the light of Crown copyright (Q2190). The DHSS and the NHRA should safeguard the

right of academics to publish research commissioned from them, subject only to legitimate delay in order to safeguard intellectual property rights.

These concerns led the government to respond (paragraph 2.25):[12]

> The Select Committee raised the issue of the publication of research funded by the Department of Health. The Government encourages the publication of research commissioned by DH, and has undertaken that the Secretary of State's consent to publication shall not be unreasonably withheld. In addition the Government has given a commitment to review DH contract conditions early in 1990 if by then there is sufficient evidence that the provisions about publication are damaging research. Directors of Department funded research units have accepted the Department's assurance on this matter and no consent to publish has been withheld since the research contract conditions were revised in 1987.

In HSR, as in any other form of research, freedom to publish is of great importance and this was considered and accepted at the inception of the discipline. That HSR can on occasion provide unwelcome findings must be accepted but administrators, managers and policy-makers continue to be sensitive to this issue. It seems strange that, although our Western democracies proclaim freedom of speech as a fundamental principle, this may still be questioned in this context. It is absolutely vital for a rigorous research discipline that integrity is maintained and that results can be published even when critical or controversial.

ACHIEVEMENTS

The total amount of grants received from the Department of Health by the St Thomas' Research Unit in 20 years was about £5 655 000 (the equivalent of £12 164 000 today). Additional sums were received from the Department of Health for specific studies as well as grants from the Medical Research Council and other research bodies. In addition to these amounts, the Medical School and Hospital resources provided support in terms of accommodation and services as well as the salaries of the core university staff including the Professor and Honorary Director of the Unit.

So was this not inconsiderable amount of public money well spent and did it provide information that improved the health of the population or the performance of the health service? Using the St Thomas' research as an example, I claim that it was and it did.

In economic terms our work on screening stands out. The trial in general practice over a ten-year period, published in 1977,[9] showed that there was little benefit of introducing multiphasic screening into the NHS. Its introduction would have increased NHS costs by at least 10 per cent each year. Over the next 30 years the savings probably amounted to more than the entire R&D budget during the period. Only in 2009 has the Department of Health succumbed to populist political pressure to introduce 'health checks' in general practice – using only economic modelling as evidence.

It is more difficult to demonstrate the worth of other HSR studies in such concrete terms and to prove without doubt their influence on policy. But our study of the effect of changes in nutritional policy in the 1970s and the establishment of the National Study of Health and Growth did undoubtedly have an influence. It was used by the then Secretary of State to reverse Labour Party policy and prevent the Labour Government from reintroducing free school milk for primary schoolchildren in 1976. The study had shown that the absence of free school milk did not harm the health of schoolchildren and could prevent the growing problem of over-nutrition (Chapter 6).

This study also demonstrated how research findings can be ignored – either through lack of understanding, knowledge or even political or administrative unwillingness to accept unwelcome findings. Started in the early 1970s, the National Study of Health and Growth was showing by the mid-1980s that the problem of obesity and being overweight in schoolchildren was increasing. If action had been taken at that time it is possible that some of the current problems of being overweight and obese could have been avoided or at least mitigated.

Our studies on health service organisation and configuration in Frimley and Basingstoke (Chapter 6), together with several other studies in the UK and elsewhere, demonstrated that change from institutional to community care was feasible and effective. The studies on the determination of health care needs in Lambeth illustrated the ability of research to illuminate a problem and to identify that a particular group of the population – the disabled – were not receiving adequate care. These studies also highlighted the need to develop a research base in general practice that could then be used for further investigations. These studies, although not unique, contributed to knowledge that was used for improvements in services and health policy.

That individual pieces of HSR rarely lead to a direct or immediate effect on policy is well illustrated by our studies on smoking (Chapter 6). The research described was among the first to show that, in the first year of life, parents' smoking was associated with an increase in respiratory illness in the child. Only one other study, published shortly before ours, had shown an association with maternal smoking habits.[13] These and later studies led to the concern with passive smoking as a health hazard. But only when passive smoking was associated with the development of lung cancer did governments begin to introduce policies to limit this damage.

Our studies on the factors involved in the take-up of smoking by schoolchildren and the harmful effects of smoking by children contributed to knowledge for the development of health promoting interventions. The trial of low-tar cigarettes demonstrated that such a strategy was not effective in reducing damage. All these studies contributed to the wider body of intelligence and knowledge required to develop appropriate methods of reducing the harm of cigarette smoking.

Those charged with developing research policy and funding research must understand the timescale and resources required. The studies on smoking in the Unit at St Thomas' started in the early 1960s and continued for the next 30 years. It was only because of the continuity of the research funding and infrastructure that this research could use the considerable expertise of the investigators and enable them to develop questions based on findings of research in different populations.

This point is illustrated again by our research on avoidable mortality (Chapter 6). Our studies showed a six-fold or greater variation in standardised mortality ratios for a few selected conditions – such as appendicitis, acute respiratory infection in young children, Hodgkin's Disease, tuberculosis, chronic rheumatic heart disease, maternal deaths – between different areas in England. The conditions had been chosen on the accepted basis that few, if any, deaths should occur with the current state of medical practice.

This work, undertaken from the early 1980s and based on research published in the US at the end of the 1970s, was taken up by the popular press but did not achieve any recognition from those concerned with the assessment of health service performance until 2010. The recently proposed reforms to the NHS include the use of outcome measures[14] – 30 years after completion of our work and publication of the results! McKee and Nolte,[15] who acknowledge the work at St Thomas', have apparently been able to promote the implementation better than any of the original studies.

Researchers have no problem in accepting the background role that they play and it is difficult, if not impossible, to attribute any change in health service practice or policy directly to individual research endeavours. I hope, however, that this book will help to demonstrate how HSR can illuminate and improve both health service practice and policy, and how important such research is and how much resource would be wasted in its absence.

REFERENCES

1 Medical Research Council (1948). Streptomycin in Tuberculosis Trials Committee. Streptomycin treatment of tuberculosis. *British Medical Journal*, 2, 769–83.

2 Cochrane, A.L. (1972). *Effectiveness and Efficiency: Random Reflections on Health Services*. London: Nuffield Provincial Hospitals.

3 Garrett, S.A., Stephenson, R.L., Holland, W.W. and Roth, I.Z. (1966). The need for intensive nursing care. *British Journal of Preventive and Social Medicine*, 20, 34–41.

4 Department of Health Social Security, Report of the Resource Allocation Working Party (1976). *Sharing Resources for Health in England*. London: HMSO.

5 Dixon, J. and Glennerster, H. (1995). What do we know about fund-holding in general practice. *British Medical Journal*, 311, 727.

6 Mays, N., Wyke, S., Malbon, G. and Goodwin, N. (2001). *The Purchasing of Health Care by Primary Care Organisations. An Evaluation and Guide Future Policy*. Buckingham: Open University Press.

7 Goodwin, N. (1998). *GP Fund-holding*. In: Le Grand, J., Mays, N. and Mulligan, J-A. (eds), *Learning from the NHS Internal Market: A Review of the Evidence*. London: Kings Fund Publishing, pp. 43–68.

8 Audit Commission (1996). *What the Doctor Ordered: a Study of GP Fund-holding in England and Wales*. London: HMSO.

9 South East London Screening Group (1977). A controlled trial of multiphasic screening in middle age: results of the South-East London Screening Study. *International Journal of Epidemiology*, 6, 357–63.

10 Holland W. (2009). Periodic Health Examination – a brief history and critical assessment. *Eurohealth*, 15, 16–20.

11 House of Lords Select Committee on Science and Technology (1988). *Priorities in Medical Research: Volume 1 Report*. London: HMSO.

12 Department of Health (1989). *Priorities in Medical Research, Government Response to the Third Report of the House of Lords Select Committee on Science and Technology: 1987–88 Session*. London: HMSO.

13 Harlap, S. and Davies, A.M. (1974). Infant admissions to hospital and maternal smoking. *Lancet*, 1, 529–32.

14 Department of Health (2010). *Transparency in Outcomes – a Framework for the NHS*. London: Crown, 14481.

15 Nolte, E. and McKee, M. (2004), *Does Healthcare Save Lives? Avoidable Mortality Revisited*. London: The Nuffield Trust.

Postscript

I have tried in this account of HSR to describe a variety of topics investigated by my St Thomas' Research Unit and to assess both the successes and the failures. In a number of the issues tackled – for example, screening and resource allocation – the lessons learnt have, over time, come to be neglected or disregarded.

Although the determination by the Department of Health to fund HSR has continued, training for new researchers instituted and calls for research proposals advertised, it is depressing that two of the major issues confronting health policy recently have not been researched.

The first of these concerns the introduction of polyclinics. In 2007 a series of papers was published by the Department of Health, the Strategic Health Authority for London and the King's Fund at the instigation of Lord Darzi, a Minister of Health, with proposals designed to improve health care, particularly in London.[1–4] The nub of the proposals was the building of a number of polyclinics, usually one per 100 000 population, which would house primary care, diagnostic services and some outpatient services. These reports were prepared largely by clinicians and health service managers, and had a great deal of input from management consultants (McKinsey). Although these reports had laudable aims and tackled issues amenable to HSR, no HSR researcher was involved with the technical and analytical work. The absence of qualified, expert researchers led to a number of basic errors. Examples of these were that projections of demand were based on statistics of events, rather than on individuals treated; community care estimates were based on the statistics collected in only two Primary Care Trusts, in which there was a four-fold variation; conditions chosen for illustration of important and frequent 'long-term conditions' were based on the opinions of participating clinicians (for acute specialties) rather than on factual data – thus omitting such conditions as arthritis and back pain. In the development of models of risk factors and prevalence of coronary heart disease, smoking, ethnicity and obesity were omitted. There was little concern with mental health. These are some of the major methodological issues (although there were many more) which these reports failed to address. They were subject to criticism,[5] no notice was taken and a £100 million building project was launched to develop the polyclinics. Not unexpectedly this has now slowed down – and the practicalities and need for these polyclinics in the present straitened financial climate are being questioned.

The second issue concerns the structure of the NHS. The 2011 Coalition Government has launched a series of proposals for changing the structure of the NHS as well as of public health.[6–8] None of these major changes in structure, organisation or function have been tested and evaluated. The changes in the commissioning of health services resemble, to some extent, the fundholding of the 1989–1997 period. This was evaluated in a number of studies – and although the select group of GPs who became fundholders appreciated the opportunities, the benefits or improvements were marginal, if not non-existent.[9, 10] The changes to public health, with transfer of the function to some extent to Local Authorities resembles the situation which existed before 1974 and was not considered, at that time, to meet the needs of the twentieth century and chronic disease in particular. This change to public health, in 1974, was the result of many consultations and experiments over a period of about 12 years.[11–13]

This current evolution of change in the provision of preventive, curative and caring health services without undertaking any adequate form of HSR or reference to past publications and experience is profoundly depressing. I have deliberately chosen examples from the past New Labour and current Coalition Governments to illustrate that the neglect of HSR is not necessarily political.

It is worth speculating why HSR is neglected in situations where its expertise could be of assistance in the improvement of the health care. Time is an important issue. Both the examples quoted above were designed and implemented over a period of one to three years (so far). To have mounted new research to illuminate either of the two topics – polyclinics, change in commissioning – would probably have taken one to two years to design and pilot, at least one year to run and a further period of one to two years to analyse the results and discuss the findings – that is, somewhat longer than the introduction and implementation of a new structure or service without the needed HSR. Under our system of adversarial government, this kind of time frame is rarely possible. This implies that in order for HSR to be used in such instances party political issues cannot be involved. If we have more coalition governments it might be possible to achieve the researchers' dream that research on profoundly 'political' issues, such as the structure and function of the NHS, can be mounted. But researchers must also appreciate that some issues are of a deeply ideological nature – for example, rationing of health care, purchasing of health care, planning. It is unlikely that politicians will be courageous enough to research such issues objectively – the hope has to be that they will be willing to learn from past experience and take note of former successes and failures. Unfortunately lessons from history are rarely remembered or taken into account by those responsible for policy – whether politicians or administrators. This is true not only for health or social policy, but also in other areas such as foreign affairs or finance. In addition, researchers must accept, however unwillingly, the effect popular opinion, the media or 'common sense' has on health policy. Thus most lay people consider preventive (periodic health) examinations (MOTs) worthwhile – even if they have been shown to be ineffective in improving health.[14]

It is also difficult to see how the temptation for policy-makers (political or administrative) to make changes on the basis of their own or their friends' experiences or feelings, or of media pressures, can be avoided or resisted.

Even if current events are profoundly depressing for those of us involved in HSR, it is vital that the health service researchers continue to undertake appropriate studies and do not attempt to cut corners to make a study politically acceptable or reduce their willingness to tackle difficult issues.

If politicians, civil servants, health service managers and their advisers would spend the resources that are and have been expended on management consultancy, there would be a far greater ability to expand HSR, sustain more academic training in the discipline and enable the HSR capacity to be adequate to answer questions posed in a timely manner. Of course, for the commissioners there would be the disadvantages of the need to formulate precise questions, results that might challenge and even contradict their opinions and attitudes, and far less money would be spent on answering health policy questions since academics earn less than management consultants!

REFERENCES

1 Darzi, Professor Lord (2007). *Healthcare for London: A Framework for Action*. London: NHS.
2 Darzi, Professor Lord (2007). *Healthcare for London: A Framework for Action. 2nd Edition*. London: NHS.
3 Department of Health (2007). *Our NHS, Our Future. NHS Next Stage Review*. October. London: Department of Health.
4 Healthcare for London: A Framework for Action. Technical Paper. 2007.
5 Holland, W.W. (2008). Healthcare for London: a framework for action. *Clinical Medicine*, **78**, 152–4.

6 Department of Health (2010). *Equity and Excellence: Liberating the NHS.* London: Department of Health.

7 Department of Health (2010). *Healthy Lives, Healthy People: Our Strategy for Public Health in England.* London: Department of Health.

8 McKee, M., Hurst, L., Aldridge, R.W., Raine, R., Mindell, J.S., Wolfe, I. and Holland, W.W. (2011). Public health in England: an option for the way forward. *Lancet*, **378**(9790), 536–9.

9 Audit Commission (1996). *What the Doctor Ordered: a Study of General Practitioner Fundholders in England and Wales.* London: HMSO.

10 Le Grand, J., Mays, N. and Mulligan, J. (eds) (1998). *Learning from the NHS Internal Market. A Review of the Evidence.* London: King's Fund.

11 McLachlan, G. (ed.) (1971). *Challenges for Change. Essays on the Next Decade in the NHS.* Published for the Nuffield Provincial Hospitals Trust. Oxford and London: Oxford University Press.

12 Kember, T. and Macpherson, G. (1994). *The NHS – a Kaleidoscope of Care – Conflicts of Service and Business Values.* London: Nuffield Provincial Hospitals Trust, London.

13 McLachlan, G. (1992). *A History of the Nuffield Provincial Hospitals Trust 1940–1990.* London: Nuffield Provincial Hospitals Trust, London.

14 Holland, W.W. (2009). Periodic health examination – a brief history and critical assessment. *Eurohealth*, **15**, 16–20.

Appendix: Department of Health reports on health services research

The Department of Health reported to Parliament annually on its research. I have extracted some of the early reports on Department-funded research activities before analysing those on HSR more thoroughly.

ANNUAL REPORT ON DEPARTMENTAL RESEARCH AND DEVELOPMENT 1973

Department of Health and Social Security. London: HMSO.

This was the first formal report produced by the Department on its research activities. It states that there were 700 or so projects current in the central programme.

> In the health field there is a very long tradition of government support for medical research. The main channel for it has been the Medical Research Council, the MRC, but the former Ministry of Health collaborated with the MRC in support of research in public health laboratories, itself promoted ad hoc projects from a very early date, and from 1958, operated through hospital boards, a scheme of decentralised clinical research. This scheme is now running at a level of 1¼ million pounds per annum, covering some 1200 projects.

The volume of centrally promoted medical research began to increase in the early part of the last decade as the rapid post-Second World War advances in science and technology generally called for reassessment and application in the service of new ideas, techniques and equipment. In 1963–1964, the Ministry of Health began to reserve special funds for clinical research and to set up a medical research administrative organisation. The following year it established the nucleus of a scientific and technical organisation and provided funds for the technical assessment and development of medical equipment and appliances. In 1961 the Ministry of Health had also formed a division to examine problems of management, particularly in the hospitals, and to pursue good practice norms. This division included staff concerned with budgeting, organisation and methods, building and engineering practice and supplies. It also collected and disseminated information on innovations in hospital practice, and in 1963, secured funds for operational research in aid of the service.

The following year, provision was made for similar 'operational' research in the other parts of the NHS, while a professional administrative group was organised with finance for the planning of R&D and hospital building and engineering. Subsequently, in 1967, an experimental NHS computer programme was launched. It is stated that direct research by departments was stimulated as well as research through the Social Science Research Council (SSRC), but springing from a much less well-developed base. Progress in social research relating to the Ministry's former welfare functions and those in childcare, assumed from the Home Office, was much less rapid than in medicine, as can be seen in the balance of the present programme. In 1964–1965, the Ministry was supporting pockets of research with an estimated expenditure of £40 000 for clinical research, £100 000 for operational research and £100 000 for equipment and appliances in building research, as well as the decentralised clinical research scheme for £400 000. By 1967–1968 it had added two more – namely an internal social science research unit and a group dealing with the application of computers to hospital administration and patient management – and the scale of operations had reached £1¾ million. The Ministry consolidated these activities by establishing a research division, which, jointly with a section of the medical staff, became responsible for the management of all research, except for that in equipment and engineering and building which remained separate for technical reasons.

A Departmental R&D Committee was set up. The Department now had in-house research, or research related resources, in statistics; social sciences; management services; operational research and relating to artificial limbs and appliances; and bio-engineering. It also commissioned R&D from other governmental establishments, particularly in the scientific and technological fields, and supported research in NHS hospitals and in public health laboratories, The greater part of its programme was nevertheless carried out under arrangements with universities and other independent research institutions. These arrangements were broadly of three kinds – research units, programmed research, and specifically commissioned projects.

The units were research establishments set up specifically for research in DHSS interests in defined subject areas or specialisms. They differed from Research Council or in-house units in that the staff were not employed by the Department and the support contracts were for specified periods of five or seven years, and were subject to review and renewal or extension on mutual satisfaction. They had a common feature with Research Council units that the arrangements focused on the Directors and could be terminated on their leaving or retirement. The programme of work and the budgets of units were settled, usually annually, with the Department, directly, or through a steering committee. Research to be carried out arose on the unit's own initiative, or on referral by the Department, or more commonly, out of the dialogue between the researchers and the Department's research administrative and policy divisions. Whatever the origins, the research was designed by the unit and was subject to approval on the criteria of relevance to service interest in 'scientific sciences'.

There were 30 such units providing specialisms covering a large part of the DHSS range of interests – for example, the epidemiology of disease; medical engineering; psychiatry; human nutrition; food science; childcare and development; cancer epidemiology; chronic disease control; rehabilitation; social work; mental handicap; drug and alcohol addiction; nursing; information science; the problems of aging and so on.

The purpose of the programmed research was to provide the opportunity and stimulus for sustained and coordinated research related to service objectives to bring the researcher into closer contact with the policy-makers and service administrators and vice versa. The latter relationship associated the researcher with the testing and application of research results. Arrangements were made with existing establishments for support of a series of research projects over a period usually of between three and five years, such as, for example, for a series of sample studies on a recorded population, or a programme of development in dental materials. The programme was submitted at the invitation of the Department or spontaneously, but in neither case was it required to be sufficiently descriptive of its scope and methods to be referred, if the Department thought appropriate, to independent assessors. Separate projects undertaken under the programme were subject to specific approval and the programme as a whole was reviewed periodically. The purpose of this type of commission, as of the units, was to provide a more sustained and comprehensive study in important problem areas. The arrangements differed from those for the units in that the group was not constituted specifically for DHSS research purposes. The scale of support was usually somewhat less, and the Directors did not enjoy such close relationships with departmental and health and social service staff. There were 40 such programmes.

The third and basic research instrument was the self-contained commissioned research project. Research projects could originate as spontaneous proposals from outside the Department or as a departmental initiative. The Department reserved a proportion of its research funds for the support of such spontaneous proposals which nevertheless were judged on the criteria of relevance, from service interests, and scientific merit. This facility was important as a source of fresh talent and ideas for the wider programme and as a symbol of the open-mindedness of the Department to independent enquiry into its work. There were 500 single projects with this type of support, mainly of up to three years' duration.

All research had a designated customer who was a senior officer with relevant policy interest. The sponsors were responsible for the decision that research be undertaken in their fields and ultimately for the application of the results. Professional and administrative research staff advised the sponsors on the scientific and technical aspects of the research to develop research resources to meet the sponsors' needs, to arrange for the assessment of proposals, to draw up and place contracts, and to make the necessary arrangements for the monitoring of progress and reports. Project or liaison officers were appointed to all projects. The committee itself authorised overall financial allocations and major projects. Since the issue of the 1971 *White Paper Framework for Government Research and Development*, Command 5046, the Department appointed a Chief Scientist in supporting scientific organisation and made new arrangements to give greater effect to the principles of research management outlined in the White Paper. Under these arrangements a team of scientists had been appointed on a part-time basis, and formed in 1971 the Chief Scientist Research Committee (CSRC), chaired by the Chief Scientist. One of the tasks for this Committee was to consider the R&D programme as a whole and to put forward advice through the Chief Scientist to the Department's planning committee. The arrangements also provided for the strengthening, in collaboration between all concerned, in the formulation, management and implementation of the R&D programme, by bringing together informal liaison groups in the appropriate areas:

- The departmental divisions of all disciplines responsible for the development of the services.
- The Chief Scientist's advisers whose role is essentially to ensure that the programme was subject to scientific scrutiny as to feasibility, quality and assessment of results.
- The research management branches which were responsible for the translation of research objectives into a sound, manageable and consistent programme of R&D.

- The research contractors including the Research Council who would carry out the research.

The arrangements were designed to allow all four contributors to play their proper role in a constructive way. Further, each member of the CSRC also served as an adviser on one or more of several specialist groups dealing with major parts of the R&D programme. These were: HSR board; personal social services group; departmental social security research policy; the advisory committee on the application of computers in the NHS; the departmental supply and equipment R&D committee; the departmental building working party; and the panel of medical research. Responsibilities of the Chief Scientist and those bodies appointed to support the post related to the organisation of R&D in England and Wales; Scotland had its own organisation.

The scale of the Department's R&D programme grew from an expenditure of £8 million pounds in 1971–1972 to £16 million pounds in 1973–1974. Of this, £3.3 million was spent on units in 1971, £4.2 million in 1972–1973 and £5.9 million in 1973–1974. The Department gave breakdowns on expenditure on individual subjects which were grouped together, such as for example, surveillance and maintenance of population health standards – for example, nutrition; environment and various public heath investigations; development of health and social care services; specific vulnerable subject groups, particularly service sectors; and so on. The headings assigned to research projects were somewhat arbitrary.

The Report gives a reasonable description of the major projects and programmes of research and major topics covered, such as, for example, the establishment of a cancer epidemiology unit under Sir Richard Doll at Oxford. Needs, such as problems of research in stroke and in cardiovascular disease, were also identified. Since these were of such importance, great play was made that something needed to be done. It is of interest that this official account of HSR funded by the Department differs in its description and evaluation of organisation and effectiveness from that described earlier in the book – which is a more historical analysis.

DHSS HANDBOOK OF RESEARCH AND DEVELOPMENT 1979

Department of Health and Social Security. London: HMSO.

Professor Arthur Buller took over responsibility as Chief Scientist from Sir Douglas Black in August 1978. He retained an advisory role in relationship to the research programme for NHS computer supplies, building and engineering, but he took full administrative responsibility for the Office of the Chief Scientist (OCS). This was reorganised to provide him with more effective support. The previous administrative and medical branches of R&D were brought within the OCS and social work and nursing research remained accountable to their own professional heads but responsible to the Chief Scientist for that part of their work concerned with the research. In addition, there was the establishment of Departmental Research Strategy Committee under the chairmanship of the Chief Scientist. The Chief Scientist reported direct to the Permanent Secretary and also had a seat on the departmental committees concerned with service strategy and priorities for Health and Personal Social Services (HPSS) and Social Security. The Chief Scientist's Research Committee met in April 1978 and was then disbanded since the new Chief Scientist's role and responsibility left it without a clear function. Scientific advice was available to the Chief Scientist both from his own staff and external advisers. Almost 100 scientific advisers helped the Chief Scientist in this task, and a meeting of all his advisers was held in March 1979. This afforded the opportunity for a useful exchange of views involving directors of research units and programmes. Research liaison groups (RLGs) began to use ad hoc working groups to deal with specialised tasks or subjects with all the RLGs revising their strategy documents. The major problems facing the OCS remained the shortage of research management staff and the lack of positive research planning in the areas not covered by the RLGs or similar bodies. The arrangements for commissioning biomedical research were revised in April 1978. The national Health Departments now informed the Medical Research Council of their research requirements under 27 broad headings of disease and services, leading to a programme of commissioned research under the headings and on specific commissions. The value of the programme undertaken for DHSS and the Welsh Office in 1978–1979 was £10.7 million. The Report gives full details of the strategy of each of the RLGs that had been created, as well as the publications resulting from the commissioned research.

The total spend on research in 1977–1978 was £20 700 000 and in 1978–1979 was £21 997 000; HSR was £4 400 000 in 1978–1979; the Medical Research Council spend was £8 900 000 in 1977–1978 and £10 700 000 in 1978–1979.

DHSS HANDBOOK OF RESEARCH AND DEVELOPMENT 1981

Department of Health and Social Security. London: HMSO.

During 1981 there were further reductions in the number of staff in the OCS because of the cuts in civil service manpower. New arrangements were designed to consolidate in a more economic and effective way the interaction between the Medical Research Council and HSR. The Health Departments and the Medical Research Council agreed that the commissioning funds would be transferred back to the science budget on the understanding that the Medical Research Council:

> would continue to meet the needs and priorities of the health departments in the Council's programme of biomedical research, and will also undertake to mount and manage in partnership with the Department of Health and Social Security some HSR, on the basis of agreed administrative and financial arrangements.

The Health Departments continued to maintain a close interest in the biomedical research undertaken by the Medical Research Council. The Chief Medical Officers of the DHSS and the Scottish Home and Health Department as well as the Chief Scientist were full members of the Medical Research Council boards. Other Health Department officials were allowed to attend as observers. The Health Departments nominated three independent scientific members to each of the three Medical Research Council boards. The Medical Research Council, it was agreed, should engage in HSR to a greater extent, in Medical Research Council units and by grant support to universities. The agreed aim was to increase, over time, that part of the base of HSR provided by the Medical Research Council, so the Council could also undertake commissions for such research in a customer–contractor relationship through the DHSS. The DHSS accepted that further development of the base for HSR depended in part on the emergence of suitable workers in the field and the establishment of new Medical Research Council units as a matter for the Council. Medical Research Council HSR was to be jointly monitored by the Council and DHSS.

Total spend in 1979–1980 was £25 083 000 and in 1980–1981 was £30 756 000. Of this, HSR received £4 865 000 and £5 784 000 respectively; the Medical Research Council received £11 400 000 and £13 700 000 in these two years.

DHSS HANDBOOK OF RESEARCH AND DEVELOPMENT 1982

Department of Health and Social Security. London: HMSO.

Professor Buller ended his period as Chief Scientist on 31 July 1981 and was succeeded in a part-time capacity by Sir Desmond Pond, Professor of Psychiatry at the London Hospital, from March 1982. The post of Deputy Chief Scientist and Controller of R&D was created. And it was noted that the Medical Research Council decided to set up a health service research panel. The expenditure on research was presented in a somewhat different form in this Report – social security and health services were grouped together and were in 1981–1982, £13 800 000 and in 1982–1983, £13 100 000. Total research spend was £22 800 000 in 1981–1982 and £22 500 000 in 1982–1983.

DHSS HANDBOOK OF RESEARCH AND DEVELOPMENT 1983

Department of Health and Social Security. London: HMSO.

Professor Robin Cole joined the Department as Deputy Chief Scientist and Controller of R&D from the Laboratory of Developmental Genetics at Sussex University in August 1982. Research spent in 1982–1983 totalled £22 680 000 and in 1983–1984, £19 130 000; health and personal social services/social security (HPSS/SS) totalled £13 100 000 in 1982–1983 and £11 500 000 in 1983–1984.

DHSS HANDBOOK OF RESEARCH AND DEVELOPMENT 1984

Department of Health and Social Security. London: HMSO.

Expenditure on research in 1983–1984 totalled £19 600 000 and in 1984–1985, £18 580 000; HPSS/SS totalled £11 500 000 in 1983–1984 and £11 100 000 in 1984–1985.

DHSS HANDBOOK OF RESEARCH AND DEVELOPMENT 1985

Department of Health and Social Security. London: HMSO.

Sir Desmond Pond completed his three-year term of appointment of Chief Scientist in 1985 and Professor Cole continued in his post as Deputy Chief Scientist and Controller of Research. Research expenditure in 1984–1985 totalled £18 700 000 and in 1985–1986, £20 020 000; HPSS/SS totalled £11 050 000 in 1984–1985 and £11 480 000 in 1985–1986.

DHSS HANDBOOK OF RESEARCH AND DEVELOPMENT 1986

Department of Health and Social Security. London: HMSO.

Professor Francis O'Grady took on the post of Chief Scientist on 1 September 1986. Professor Cole left the Department in December 1985 and was succeeded as Director of Research Management and Deputy Chief Scientist by Dr Jeremy Metters on 10 March 1986. The Division's title changed from the OCS to the Research Management Division. Research expenditure in 1985–1986 totalled £20 450 000 and in 1986–1987, £22 460 000; HPSS/SS totalled £11 351 000 in 1985–1986 and £11 758 000 in 1986–1987.

DHSS HANDBOOK OF RESEARCH AND DEVELOPMENT 1987

Department of Health and Social Security. London: HMSO.

For the first time the Report stated that the DHSS had priorities. These were: health and personal social services; acquired immune deficiency syndrome; demands and effect on and effectiveness of acute sector services; the transition to community care; consumer attitudes to the health and personal social services; influencing of lifestyles – for example, in relation to drug abuse, professional manpower, and for social security; the transition to community care; and evaluation of the effectiveness of social programmes. Research expenditure in 1986–1987 totalled £23 195 000 and in 1987–1988, £25 904 000; HPSS/SS totalled £12 664 000 in 1986–1987 and £14 614 000 in 1987–88.

DHSS HANDBOOK OF RESEARCH AND DEVELOPMENT 1988

Department of Health and Social Security. London: HMSO.

The philosophy in this Report was that:

- Assessment is an activity integral to the functioning of those associated with the management of the programme and is a task carried out by all personnel.
- *Advice is taken from independent scientific and service referees by a peer review*, and from practitioners actively involved in the matter of the study.
- The outcome measures used for the assessment of research have been designed to identify and document research strategies and activities that are most relevant to the Department, often utilising performance indicators for research that have been developed for other purposes. They have the support of the Departmental Research Committee.
- The assessment of R&D is commonly a matter of judgement, wherever possible hard data are used, but there are research situations where numerical data are not available, and if generated, have only a subjective basis.

Current Assessment Procedures

These are exercised by the Departmental Research Committee, the Chief Scientist and his advisers, the divisions responsible for research management and the policy divisions. The Chief Scientist's functions include giving advice and guidance on scientific feasibility and validity.

Assessment of Research Units

The Chief Scientist conducts periodic reviews of all DHSS centrally funded research units. During these visits the Chief Scientist is accompanied by independent advisers who help the Chief Scientist in the assessment.

Assessment of Individual Projects

The divisions responsible for management of individual units, programmes and so on use the following criteria.

Prior to funding:
1. Relevance.
2. Degree of customer support; clear indication of use which will be made of the results.
3. Quality of study, design and methodology.
4. Identification of targets for phase completion; monitoring during the study.
5. Standard of conduct of work.
6. Maintenance of timetable.
7. Maintenance of interim objectives specified to the outside.

On completion of the work:
1. Completion on schedule and within cost allocation.
2. Degree of relevance to customer's needs.
3. Contribution to knowledge of the subject.
4. Utility of the findings directly or indirectly.
5. Value for money.

Ex Ante Assessments

All projects and programmes are judged on three criteria:

1. Whether the research relates closely to ministerial requirements and therefore to policy interests.
2. Whether the work is scientifically sound.
3. Whether the work is expected to be good value for money, in turn, appraisal monitoring.

All projects and programmes have an identified manager or liaison officer in the DHSS whose task is to ensure the work progresses adequately. In addition to close monitoring the progression and targets by the liaison officer, some studies are subject to other assessment mechanisms, such as annual reports, peer review and customer visits.

Ex Post Appraisal

Reports and output from research are assessed for quality and relevance both by in-house staff and by independent assessors. The outcome of these assessments will determine the use subsequently made of the research results as a basis for policy.

Selection and Assessment of Research

New work is introduced into the programme through a process in which policy divisions are required to bid for funds for projects within themes set by the Departmental Research Committee. Once bids have been received within these themes, in-house meetings of officials are held to prioritise them. Criteria vary but usually include ministerial priority, necessity of research to inform policy action, precision of a specification, intrinsic value of project, relation to other relevant work in the field, readiness to go. Once a project has been selected, detailed planning is undertaken by the research managers and the policy division working together either with an ad hoc committee or an existing committee. The brief is then tendered. Competitive tendering is used where possible but low cost is not the only criterion used for selection. Each research project has to fulfil three criteria of scientific quality, policy relevance and value for money. Once underway, the study is subjected to regular scrutiny.

DEPARTMENT OF HEALTH YEARBOOK OF RESEARCH AND DEVELOPMENT 1990

Department of Health. London: HMSO.

Total expenditure for R&D was £60 100 000 of which £21 100 000 was for outside work. HPSS received £15 400 000.

Priorities for Commissioned Research

Acute hospital sector-based services needs and respective selected illnesses – for example: cancer; cardiovascular illness; finance; organisational quality of acute sector hospital services and evaluation of the effectiveness and cost effectiveness of clinical procedures; drugs and equipment; AIDS; childcare; research into adequacy and cost-effectiveness of services for children under five years and children in need of care and protection; community care and development of community care for elderly people; primary health care; research into the planning and provision of effective, efficient and acceptable primary health care; public health; research into the prevention of disease prolonging life and promoting health; priorities into research concerning food safety, nutrition, environmental pollution and clinical disease; workforce; research into education, training, recruitment, retention, remuneration and effective deployment of staff.

A major development in 1989–1990 was the announcement that the Department intended to appoint a Chief of Research and Development, now renamed Director of Research and Development. This Report contains a chapter by Frances O'Grady who finished his term of appointment in 1990. O'Grady said that the objective of the Department's research programme was to support ministers and policy development, but its critics claim that it should have been supporting clinical and operational needs of service provision.

Index